PRACTICAL YOGA NIDRA

PRACTICAL
YOGA
NIDRA

A 10-STEP METHOD
to REDUCE STRESS, IMPROVE SLEEP,
and RESTORE YOUR SPIRIT

SCOTT MOORE

ROCKRIDGE
PRESS

Interior and Cover Designer: Tricia Jang
Photo Art Director/Art Manager: Hillary Frileck
Editor: Lauren Ladoceour
Production Editor: Ashley Polikoff
Production Manager: Riley Hoffman
Photography: Author photo © Alex Adams

ISBN: Print 978-1-64611-028-5 | eBook 978-1-64611-029-2

R0

To all my teachers, especially
SENECA, ELIO, AND LIAM,
where love is everything
and everything is YES.

Contents

Welcome

I'm so happy you've found *Practical Yoga Nidra.* Thank you
for beginning this journey with me. This book is a product of
more than a decade of study, practice, and teaching Yoga Nidra.
This ancient practice is experiencing a renaissance today, and it's
catching on all over the world. This book is designed to help you
understand what Yoga Nidra is and give you an easy-to-follow,
10-step guide to the practice that you can start using right now to
help you reduce stress, improve sleep, and restore your spirit.

The practice of Yoga Nidra is simply about being present and
aware. It differs from most meditation styles with its emphasis on
relaxation. The roots of Yoga Nidra date back to 700 to 1,000 BCE
in India, and over the centuries its teachings have expanded from
a dualist philosophy (things being either/or) to a non-dualist philosophy (things being both/and), which you'll come to understand
as you read on.

During my very first Yoga Nidra experience, I asked myself
this essential question: "So what? What does this ancient practice mean to the modern person who wakes up every day, gets
their kids off to school, and zips off to work with a piece of toast

in hand?" It took many years of asking this question to find an answer, but along the way, I've learned how Yoga Nidra can be a beautiful and fascinating method of self-discovery and that it can be very practical in the twenty-first century, just as it was thousands of years ago. It helps us solve the same essential human problem: feeling separate from Source (aka the Universe, God, or Creation). For me, Yoga Nidra has been the most helpful, profound, and relaxing method for facilitating reunification—that *yoking*—with my essential being. I'm ecstatic to share my experience and knowledge with you in a way that's easy to understand and practice.

For many years I've been teaching Yoga Nidra and have helped people practice reconnecting with their essential being, their True Self. Hopefully this book will demystify the practice of Yoga Nidra and help you use this powerful tool in a way that is practical and real for you without dumbing it down or denigrating its tradition. In fact, I believe that the power of yoga and Yoga Nidra in part lies in the fact that they are adaptable to the needs of the person who practices them, whether that's in the year 20 BCE or 2020 CE.

Because Yoga Nidra is the practice of learning to engage with our ultimate being, you'll notice that superlative concepts are often designated with capital letters to emphasize their spiritual or magnanimous quality. So expect to see capitalized words and phrases like True Self, True Nature, Beingness, Awareness, Both/And nature, Source, and Self throughout this book. All these words are emphasized in a way that helps designate them as the eternal part of our being.

I invite you to be open to the teachings of this book. I believe these simple steps have the potential to change your life for the better and ultimately help you become a more whole, complete, and happy version of yourself. My sincere desire is that through these 10 steps, you uncover what was there all along: your limitless, loving, and whole True Self.

CHAPTER ONE

TAP INTO THE
POWER OF
YOGA NIDRA

What Is Yoga Nidra?

Yoga Nidra means "the yoga of sleep," but don't let the name fool you. In truth, this ancient practice is more about learning to wake up. *Nidra* refers to that daydream state between wakefulness and sleep. Think of the paradox of sleeping wakefulness as a bridge between otherwise disparate elements, such as consciousness and unconsciousness, spirit and form, and the ego-self and the True Self.

Yoga Nidra is essentially a guided meditation during which the practitioner usually lies down, closes their eyes, and becomes very relaxed as they are guided by a facilitator into deeper and deeper layers of relaxed Awareness. By recording the scripts in this book and playing them back, you will be both the facilitator and the practitioner.

A Yoga Nidra practice often lasts between 10 and 45 minutes, during which time the facilitator guides the practitioner systematically into a focused but neutral observation of the five koshas (or sheaths, which you can think of as layers over your True Self). These are the objects of the ego as well as physical sensations, thoughts, and emotions. The method's aim is to help you learn to stop identifying with the ego-self by peeling back the koshas like layers of skin off an onion and instead identify with the core of your True Nature—pure Awareness. It's like napping your way to enlightenment!

While not everyone emerges from every practice having "seen the light," it's incredible how many people report experiencing massive benefits, even after their first session. Rather than tell my students the benefits of the practice, I allow the practice to speak for itself. I typically start a Yoga Nidra class by asking return students how they benefit from the practice. Eager hands shoot into the air as students happily report a wide array of benefits, including lowered stress, being less reactive, greater happiness, better sleep, lowered blood pressure, less anxiety and depression, more energy, accelerated learning, increased creativity, higher performance and productivity, general well-being, better digestion, greater optimism, spiritual insight, confidence, and a grounded sense of purpose, clarity, and optimism.

In more extreme cases, I've personally used Yoga Nidra, often in tandem with a licensed clinical therapist, as a powerful tool to help people who suffer from issues like PTSD, trauma, sexual abuse, chronic anxiety and depression, eating disorders, alcohol and chemical dependency, and chronic and terminal illnesses better cope with their issues. I have also used Yoga Nidra to maximize the performance of world-class artists, including the cast of the Broadway show STOMP, Justin Timberlake's dancers and backup singers, and the dancers of Ballet West. I've trained top-level athletes to use Yoga Nidra to help them perform and win ultramarathons, ultra-cycling events, and Olympic events.

I've even trained high school kids to use Yoga Nidra to conquer test anxiety. At one of my recent trainings, I taught a marriage and family lawyer how to use Yoga Nidra with her clients to help them manage divorce proceedings as calmly and civilly as possible.

The benefits of Yoga Nidra have also been tested in clinical studies. Currently, Yoga Nidra teachers, such as clinical psychologist Dr. Richard C. Miller, are conducting scientific studies to show how it can benefit war veterans in prisons and hospitals. A report in the *Journal of Caring Sciences* shows Yoga Nidra to be a successful therapy to help with anxiety, depression, positive well-being, general health, and vitality scores as well as hormonal levels associated with menstrual irregularity.

So how can a practice of simply lying down and being guided through something like a body scan or an examination of your thoughts provoke such remarkable benefits? The idea is that when you're aligned with your True Self through—and as—deep Awareness, you experience the part of you that is always perfect. More simply, as you experience yourself as Awareness, you experience wholeness. In such wholeness, there's nothing you can't do or be. Wholeness means healed. All the benefits my students call out in class are merely the by-products of wholeness.

One of the essential truths I love about yoga and Yoga Nidra is the idea that these practices don't give you anything you don't have already. Rather, they help you remove the layers that conceal your fundamental wholeness, a wholeness that has always been and will always be. Experiencing this wholeness boils down to Awareness, and Yoga Nidra is a very relaxing yet powerful way to develop your Awareness.

The 10-Step Method

The 10-step method in this book is designed to be the most streamlined and practical guide to helping you learn how to practice Yoga Nidra and reap its vast benefits. It systematically deepens your Awareness through increasingly subtle layers. By following this method, you will begin an effective Yoga Nidra practice starting on day one. It offers you essential, detailed, and simple instructions on how and why to do the practice as well as scripts, so there's no guesswork about how to practice. Each chapter provides you with a short and long Yoga Nidra meditation script. You will record these scripts on your smartphone or other device and play them back, thereby leading yourself into a deep Yoga Nidra practice. Here are the 10 steps:

STEP 1: SET AN INTENTION. Learn the value of setting an intention and how to start your Yoga Nidra practice with one.

STEP 2: ENTER A SAFE HAVEN. Build your mental/emotional sanctuary to establish a steady and secure ground for you to experience this profound practice and feel wonderful in the process.

STEP 3: SCAN THE BODY. Use an effective body scan to establish a keen awareness while calming and activating certain functions of your brain and nervous system.

STEP 4: FOLLOW THE BREATH. Move your awareness into the subtle body through awareness of breath and energy.

STEP 5: TURN TOWARD EMOTIONS. Experience your emotions as a gift to practice awareness rather than as something to wish for or keep at bay.

STEP 6: WITNESS THOUGHTS. Be a witness to your thoughts and learn to stop identifying with them.

STEP 7: TAP INTO JOY. Experience a state of bliss and enter through a secret door into a joy that transcends any event or circumstance that could dictate your life.

STEP 8: OBSERVE THE SELF. Witness your Self, your Beingness, the part of you that exists independent of your body, energy, thoughts, beliefs, and emotions.

STEP 9: VISUALIZE. Use all the tools you've cultivated in your Yoga Nidra practice to visualize and achieve great sleep, reduce anxiety, and be at your best.

STEP 10: INTEGRATE YOUR PRACTICE. Bring everything together into a complete Yoga Nidra practice.

Once you've learned each of the 10 steps, you'll spend the last chapter strengthening the practice by learning to welcome your inner peace and how to customize your practice so that it can be even more powerful and personal. Throughout, I'll discuss the real-life application of Yoga Nidra and how to live your life from a place of greater Awareness, clarity, and self-knowledge afforded by your Yoga Nidra practice.

SUPPORTED SAVASANA

The asana, or pose, that traditionally facilitates Yoga Nidra practice is Savasana. The Sanskrit word means "corpse pose" in English. It offers the best opportunity for the body to relax and enter into the Nidra state, that of relaxed Awareness.

Support your Savasana with some extra props—namely blankets, bolsters, or cushions. Do this by placing your yoga mat on the floor, followed by one or two blankets, folded longways, the length of your yoga mat. Lie faceup on your blankets and place another folded blanket or pillow under your head. Tuck a rolled blanket, cushion, or pillow under your knees, especially if you have a sensitive lower back. Allow your arms to rest comfortably at your side, or place your hands on your belly. While not necessary, an eye pillow or eye mask is nice to help relax your nervous system by softening the eyes and blocking out light.

Comfort is paramount in Yoga Nidra, so if lying on the floor is unavailable or uncomfortable, feel free to lie on a bed, couch, or massage table. You may also sit in a chair. While there's nothing wrong with falling asleep in Yoga Nidra, I find that doing the practice on my bed or couch makes me snooze and thus it is more difficult to enter into the state of relaxed Awareness.

How to Use This Book

This book is meant to be a step-by-step guide; therefore, I encourage you to digest each chapter before moving on to the next. Of course, you can always go back and review previous chapters to clarify or deepen your understanding, but please read and practice each step one at a time to get the most benefit. I recommend getting a journal specifically for your Yoga Nidra practice so that you can spend time reflecting on your practice afterward and responding to the questions posed. Later in the book, you'll be asked to look back on your journal entries when customizing your Yoga Nidra practice.

As mentioned, each of the chapters has a short and a long guided Yoga Nidra script for you to read, record, and store on your device to be played back when you are ready to relax. These meditations are a simple way to lead yourself through your Yoga Nidra practices. The idea is to listen to each recording a few times on separate occasions, as your experience will be different each time. It's a good idea to use headphones while listening to block out noise and keep you more alert and attentive.

Don't worry about buying expensive recording equipment—most smartphones, tablets, laptops, and desktop computers have simple-to-use, built-in voice recorders. I record each Yoga Nidra practice I teach using the app that came with my phone. The quality is more than adequate for sharing and playing back for my own uses. You're welcome to buy a recorder or set up recording equipment on your computer, but unless you're already familiar with such technology, I encourage you to make this process as easy as possible. Anything will do so long as you can reliably play the guided transcript back while you are in Savasana.

There are a few helpful pointers to keep in mind when you make your recordings. For starters, speak slowly and clearly. Also, it's important to add 5- to 10-second pauses between sentences to allow space for cultivating awareness. If a script, for example, includes an invitation to sense your right hand, you'll want to pause after the instruction to allow your future self some time to do just that before the next instruction. At the end of the day, it's much better to be too slow in a Yoga Nidra practice than too fast. After you record a few of these scripts and listen back, you'll soon find a pace that works for you.

While some skillful teachers use music in tandem with the practice, I suggest recording your scripts without background music to avoid pulling your attention away from the practice. If you feel adding background music could really help you relax and improve your meditation, give it a try after practicing without music a few times. To signal the end of your practice, you can either count down from five or ring a bell to signal the completion of Yoga Nidra. If you intend to finish your script recording using a bell, have one handy before you start your recording.

Sometimes, people ask me if practicing Yoga Nidra is safe. The answer is, well, yes. There are no qualifications, and no previous experience with yoga or meditation is needed to lead yourself through Yoga Nidra. I love how powerful and accessible it is. Essentially, Yoga Nidra is accessing what already exists inside you by taking off the "costumes" you wear that cloud your Awareness.

These costumes are the titles we tend to identify with (like "parent," "successful," or "sick") that ultimately prevent us from experiencing our True Self and therefore our True Nature—both of which are Awareness itself.

If you experience severe depression, anxiety, psychosis, or other mental disorders, I encourage you to seek professional help and perhaps ask your therapist and/or doctor if you could go through these steps together as part of your therapy. Having said that, the 10-step method is safe to do on your own and will teach you how to establish a beautiful and expansive inner environment in which you will observe all that presents itself. A lot of stuff like memories, emotions, and thoughts may come up as the result of this introspection, and you will learn techniques for dealing with them if or when they do. Having a confidant you can talk to about your experiences is always beneficial.

In truth, there are as many ways to practice and teach Yoga Nidra as there are people practicing and teaching it. There is no perfect way to do this. However, my intention here is to use my experience to lead you through developing your own Yoga Nidra practice in a way that is effective, easy to follow, and streamlined. My hope is that through this 10-step guide, you'll find ready access to this beautiful practice in a way that helps you discover your own innate perfection and experience wholeness. Self-knowledge really isn't that complicated. Think of it as a tap on the forehead to "pay attention!" Yoga Nidra is my favorite way of learning the art of paying attention, and I hope it becomes yours as well.

CHAPTER TWO

STEP 1:
SET AN INTENTION

How to Choose a Sankalpa

The first step of the 10-step method is to set your intention. *Sankalpa* is a Sanskrit word that could most simply be translated as "intention." However, the practice of choosing your Sankalpa is a bit more involved than merely stating your intention for your Yoga Nidra practice. Your Sankalpa is like a personal mantra or a statement of truth that you repeat in your mind once or a few times as you begin your practice. I encourage you to sincerely consider what your Sankalpa will be each time you begin a Yoga Nidra practice. If there's something big in your life you feel you need, your Sankalpa could be the same each time. However, try to picture what specifically you need *today* in relationship to that desire. In other words, don't get stuck in the past with a Sankalpa that is outdated for you.

To choose your Sankalpa, it's best to pause for a moment, close your eyes, take a few deep breaths, and become present by opening to your senses. Then reflect for a few moments about what you need most in your life in the moment. Your Sankalpa might be for something practical and physical, something emotional, or something spiritual. You may even set an intention for the well-being of another person or whole group of people. Your Sankalpa doesn't have to be about something you want; rather, it could be about recognizing and appreciating what you already have.

It's important to make your Sankalpa just a simple sentence or phrase. This helps you gain clarity and focus on what you really need or want. Also, when choosing your Sankalpa, make it positive, specific, and present. Let's look a little more deeply at these three considerations next.

The Universe is one big, eternal yes. It's inviting you to merge into its path of awakening to a complete understanding of this Universal positivity—this "yes." Yoga Nidra is about aligning with your True Nature, and you can begin this essential alignment by choosing a Sankalpa that reflects universal positivity. Judith Hanson Lasater, one of my yoga teachers, once said, "What is worrying but praying for what you don't want?" In other words, focusing on something, good or bad, tends to bring about its realization. I grew up in Utah where virtually everyone mountain bikes in the summer and skis in the winter. Coaches in both sports teach beginners to look where they want to go rather than where they don't want to go to avoid veering off course. That's why when choosing a Sankalpa, you need to focus on what you want rather than on what you want to avoid. Positive, not negative.

The next consideration is specificity. Being specific when choosing your Sankalpa paints a bull's-eye for the Universe to aim for. In one short sentence, state the exact thing you want rather than sweeping generalities. Here's an example of the reverse: Once, a friend in her twenties asked the Universe for a car. Her intention was to own something with an automatic transmission and a sunroof. A week later, her family inherited a Lincoln Town

Car that indeed had both automatic transmission and a sunroof but smelled like an ashtray, was 12 feet long, and was probably older than she was. She drove that car gratefully but decided that the next time she made her automotive intentions known to the Universe, she would be sure to add that she wanted something a bit sportier and hipper.

Finally, when choosing your Sankalpa, it's essential to be present. The part of you that you're communicating your Sankalpa to understands *only* the present. Past and future are abstract concepts regulated by different parts of your brain and being. When making your Sankalpa, speak to what is rather than what isn't. This means formulating something you're searching for in present terms and focusing on where you're at, what you have, and who you are *now in relationship to where you wish to go.*

Here are a few examples of Sankalpas that you can complete and modify to help you create a positive, specific, and present intention:

"I'm on my road to . . ."
"I already have everything inside me that I need for . . ."
"The Universe is ready to give me . . ."

What This Practice Does for You

Your Sankalpa acts as a guiding star for how your journey of Yoga Nidra will unfold, what kind of awareness will be revealed, and which layers clouding your ability to experience your True Self will be removed. When you state your Sankalpa, you plant a living seed of spirit, hope, and desire inside your mind and heart as a clear and direct invitation to the Universe to reveal to you your True Self through that intention. Your Yoga Nidra practice cultivates the fertile soil for your seed of Awareness to grow and bloom.

To consider this concept more deeply, I'd like to introduce you to the Gayatri Mantra. This beautiful and ancient mantra is one of the oldest mantras known to us; it comes from the *Rig Veda*, part of a body of texts called the Vedas, dating between 1700 and 1100 BCE. The mantra illuminates how stating your Sankalpa before your Yoga Nidra practice works to help manifest that intention. Here is this mantra in Sanskrit:

oṃ bhūr bhuvaḥ suvaḥ
tatsaviturvareṇyaṃ
bhargo devasyadhīmahi
dhiyo yo naḥ prachodayāt

My favorite translation of the Gayatri Mantra comes from Donna Farhi, which she includes in her book *Bringing Yoga to Life*. It goes like this:

Everything on the earth and in the sky and in between
Is arising from one effulgent source
If my thoughts, words, and deeds reflected a complete understanding
    of this unity
I would be the peace I am seeking in this moment.

As this mantra says, if I understood the essence of all things—including myself and the thing I want—I'd understand that everything comes from the same source. Ultimately, I'd see that I'm no different from the thing I want. While this is nice to understand on a philosophical level, it will most likely take a lifetime of practice (or more lives if there are more to be had) to truly understand this truth. Yoga Nidra is a perfect way to practice coming to understand this truth by aligning with our magnificent Source.

According to Yoga Nidra philosophy, everything in the Universe is boiled down to Awareness. When you align with your basic Awareness through presence (Yoga Nidra being my favorite way to practice presence), you align with the origin of all things, including you and all that you feel separate from. Remember, Yoga Nidra is about remembering and experiencing our fundamental wholeness. This is why this is considered a practice of yoga, or "yoking" together of all things.

Your Sankalpa speaks to the eternal part of you that isn't dependent upon past or future. Therefore, planting the seed of Sankalpa in your heart and mind is like planting iris bulbs in the fall—they bloom in the spring whether or not you remember planting them. Because your Sankalpa works for your benefit, it's essential to be mindful and deliberate when choosing it, even if you can't remember it later.

As I've mentioned, the practice of Yoga Nidra is simply about being present. Starting your Yoga Nidra practice with your Sankalpa makes you very present by first taking a moment to recognize your needs and second by alerting the Universe how to best awaken you to your ultimate Awareness. You do this by practicing Awareness and an understanding that you are not separate from what you seek—yep, even if it's that hip sports car! The point is that *everything* is part of everything without exception.

This reminds me of Leonard Cohen's song "Anthem," in which the artist meditates on how through our perceived brokenness or sense of lack, we come to understand our own wholeness and illumination. We aren't perfect despite our brokenness but because of it. Stating our Sankalpa is alerting ourselves and the Universe to the avenue by which we are coming to know ourselves as perfect, whole beings.

5-MINUTE MEDITATION SCRIPT

To begin this Yoga Nidra practice, lie down, get comfortable, and take a couple of deep breaths. Open to broad awareness, without judgment, everything you're aware of in this moment. Merely invite, acknowledge, and observe whatever manifests. Remember, nothing is either good or bad—just information.

Now begin to create your Sankalpa. Create one specifically for this Yoga Nidra practice. Observe your life. Be as objective as possible and ask yourself what you most need or desire. Allow your heart to create your Sankalpa. It could be something physical, emotional, or spiritual. Be curious about what spontaneously comes to the surface. Don't intellectualize or imagine a Sankalpa. This is private and personal.

Now create a positive, specific, and present statement around this need or desire. You may choose a phrase like, "I'm on my road to . . ." and fill in the blank, or "I already have everything inside of me that I need for . . ." and fill in the blank, or "The Universe is ready to give me . . ." and fill in the blank. This statement is your Sankalpa. Repeat it in your mind a few times. Notice how it feels.

Your Sankalpa is now planted like a seed inside your mind and heart. This Yoga Nidra practice is cultivating the fertile ground for it to grow, and the Universe will manifest it to you as you continually practice presence.

As you finish your Yoga Nidra practice, feel your body on the floor. As a result of this Yoga Nidra practice, you'll go back into your life feeling more alive, in line with your True Nature, and ready to manifest your Sankalpa into your life.

When you hear me count down from five (or ring the bell), that will signal the end of the Yoga Nidra practice.

5, 4, 3, 2, 1 (or ring the bell).

Yoga Nidra is over.

Get Started

Record either the short or long meditation (or both) in this chapter. Then, pick a time to practice and a place where you can be undisturbed. You may choose to put a "Do Not Disturb—Yoga Nidra in Process" sign on the door. Let the people you live with know that unless the house is on fire, you shouldn't be disturbed during your practice. If you have pets, you may need to have a serious talk with them and let them know that you'll be unavailable for a while.

Choose a time to practice when you will be most alert. The state of being awake in relaxed awareness is optimal during this practice, but if you fall asleep, you're still practicing Yoga Nidra. While we are aiming for a waking state of relaxed awareness, the part of you that is listening to the Yoga Nidra practice is paying attention whether or not your waking consciousness is. In Yoga Nidra, you're communicating with the eternal part of you that is Source, that is Awareness itself. In many ways, Yoga Nidra acts as a bridge to get our waking conscious and thinking mind on board with our unconscious or being mind.

However, if you do tend to regularly doze off during Yoga Nidra, it may be a cue that you're not getting enough good, regular sleep. Sleep is generally very important to our well-being and is particularly important for developing the restful alertness necessary for the work we do with Yoga Nidra. I offer a number of ideas in chapter 11 for good sleep hygiene. Flip to page 113 for a quick review if you fall into this category.

Once you've chosen the place and time, arrange your Yoga Nidra "nest" with the props you'll need for a successful practice. I suggest using a yoga mat on the floor with a few folded blankets placed lengthwise on top so that you have a foundation that is solid yet comfortable. Also, tuck a folded blanket under your head and a rolled blanket or cushion under your knees, especially if you have a sensitive back. An eye pillow blocks out light and calms the nervous system, but it isn't required.

If getting on and off the floor is difficult, consider investing in a massage table to use for Yoga Nidra. If those options aren't practical, go ahead and use your bed or couch. Remember, you can do Yoga Nidra anywhere. In fact, if the only few minutes a day you have to practice Yoga Nidra is sitting in your car during your lunch break, then do that.

Before beginning your Yoga Nidra practice, try to make sure that all possible distractions are minimized; this includes putting your phone in airplane mode. But know that despite your best efforts, distractions will arise. These are to be expected and, strangely, even appreciated. During Yoga Nidra, your job is simply to invite, acknowledge, and observe whatever arises in your Awareness in the moment. For some reason the Universe is asking you to pay attention, and whether it's an emotion or a buzzing fly, it's all simply a practice of witnessing.

Reflect on Your Practice

As your Yoga Nidra practice concludes, take a moment to come back into the feeling of your body. While still lying on the floor, offer yourself a few deep breaths, remember what time of day it is, and gently open your eyes. When you're ready, roll over to one side and rest there for a few moments. Then sit up and give yourself a few more deep breaths. This is an excellent place to repeat your Sankalpa again in your mind, which will help you carry it forward into your everyday life.

As you reflect on your practice, try to remember what happened during the practice. A Yoga Nidra journal—a blank book to reflect on your practice and respond to the reflection questions—will be a valuable resource. If you don't have a blank journal, write on lined paper for now. You can tuck them into a journal you get for this purpose later.

Write down your immediate responses to the practice. I encourage you to write freely, without editing yourself, and simply get the words out without attempting to make them flowery or eloquent. Just do a word dump onto the page. You can also respond to some or all of these questions in your journal:

- Did you stay awake, or did you fall asleep? Did you find yourself drifting between waking and dreaming?

- Did you achieve a sense of relaxation, and what was that like?

⌀ What were you aware of during your practice?

⌀ Did anything arise that you weren't expecting?

⌀ What was your experience choosing your Sankalpa like?

⌀ Did you choose something expected or unexpected as your Sankalpa?

⌀ What, if any, were the spontaneous images, thoughts, memories, emotions, or physical sensations that arose as you went through the practice of creating your Sankalpa?

Remember that in Yoga Nidra practice, nothing is supposed to happen or not happen. Whatever happens, does. Again, our only job is to invite, acknowledge, and observe whatever arises in our field of awareness.

Even if you don't remember your Sankalpa because you fell asleep or feel like you couldn't think of one, there is a part of you that made one and does remember nonetheless. The work happens on a layer deeper than our conscious mind. Plus, just like a yoga practitioner might not nail a headstand on their first go, developing your Sankalpa is a practice and might take a few tries before it becomes natural. The important part is to be in the practice. This is another reason why it's nice to have the recordings of these scripts because you can practice this same meditation again later. I assure you that your experience will be different each time.

Full Meditation Script

Welcome to Yoga Nidra. Take a moment to become as comfortable as possible. Once you become comfortable, release any residual tension you may have by giving yourself a full breath in, holding it for one second, then let it out with a sigh. Repeat a few times.

Remember that there is nothing that is or is not supposed to happen; nothing is good or bad—it's all just information. Your only job is to invite, acknowledge, and observe all the information that comes to you with mild curiosity. If something that you're aware of persists, like pain, sensation, or something else that is calling for your attention, first practice merely welcoming it. Then recognize it for what it is—a sound, thought, or sensation, for example. Part of recognizing it means recognizing all the ways you are affected by that thing. Simply observe it and be the witness of it. That's all. Sometimes, you may choose to add a fourth stage, which is to respond to the message, but that is only after you've practiced merely witnessing it.

Now give yourself a moment to practice open awareness without any judgment to whatever your attention is aware of in this moment. It could be sounds, thoughts, sensations—anything. Practice welcoming, recognizing, and merely witnessing whatever it is that you're most aware of in this moment. Remember, nothing is good or bad. It's all simply information.

Now that you've established yourself as the observer, begin to create your Sankalpa, the seed of intention that you will plant in your mind and heart through this Yoga Nidra practice. In this moment, be only an observer of your life. Be as objective as possible and ask yourself what you need or desire in this moment. Open up and be curious about what spontaneously comes to the surface. Don't try to intellectualize or create anything.

Let the deep, knowing part of you speak to the part of you that is creating the Sankalpa. Remember that you can always change your Sankalpa for other practices, but merely be aware of what presents itself in this moment as a need or desire. It could be something physical or a desire or need for healing—physically, mentally, or spiritually. You may desire spiritual understanding or enlightenment. There is nothing too ordinary or too lofty to desire in your Sankalpa.

Once you have chosen what you need or desire, give yourself a moment to welcome this desire or need. Recognize all the ways in which this desire affects you: Does it conjure thoughts, emotions, or mental images? Where do you feel that need or desire in your body? Now give yourself a moment to simply witness this need or desire. As you practice Awareness around your need or desire, notice if anything about the need or desire has changed.

Now create a positive statement around this need or desire that is also specific and present. You may choose a phrase like "I'm on my road to . . ." and fill in the blank, or "I already have everything inside of me that I need for . . ." and fill in the blank, or "The Universe is ready to give me . . ." and fill in the blank. Once you've created your positive, specific, and present statement, repeat it in your mind a few times.

Now welcome your Sankalpa. Recognize all the ways it is currently affecting you: Where in your body do you feel it? What, if any, images, colors, thoughts, or memories spontaneously arise? Are there any words that arise in your Awareness as a response? Remember that your only job is to witness your Sankalpa.

Now that you've practiced being present to your Sankalpa, you've planted it as a seed inside your mind and your heart. Even if you forget what your Sankalpa was, this Yoga Nidra practice has cultivated the fertile ground for it to grow and bloom. The Universe will begin to manifest what you need and desire as you continually practice presence.

Again, feel your body as it lies on the floor. As the observer, experience yourself as Awareness feeling itself as a body. Feel yourself breathing and notice if you've been able to get relaxed during the process. If you can remember it, state your Sankalpa to yourself one more time in your mind. Because of this Yoga Nidra practice, you'll go back into your life feeling more alive and in line with your True Nature, and your Sankalpa will begin to manifest in your life in many clear and subtle ways.

When you hear me count down from five (or ring the bell), that will signal the end of the Yoga Nidra practice.

5, 4, 3, 2, 1 (or ring the bell).

Yoga Nidra is over.

CHAPTER THREE

STEP 2: ENTER A SAFE HAVEN

How to Connect to Your Inner Sanctuary

Quite simply, your Inner Sanctuary is your safe haven. This is your constant personal paradise, your "happy place," that you can quickly and easily access through visualization. Your Inner Sanctuary helps you establish a feeling of safety and a foundation of Awareness, which you will deepen, layer by layer, throughout the rest of your Yoga Nidra practice.

Feeling how you feel in your Inner Sanctuary is how your True Self feels all the time. Feeling anything else is merely illusions of the ego. I know, I know, welcome to humanity, right?

Well, practicing Yoga Nidra helps you embrace what I call your Both/And nature—your spiritual nature and your human nature together experiencing your True Nature—that which encompasses both. In truth, as a human being, the only way to experience your True Nature is through your human senses. Since the essence of your True Nature is Awareness, anything that helps you practice Awareness is a powerful tool on your path to self-discovery. Nothing helps you pay attention better and nothing is more human than your senses. They are constantly bombarding you with information, inviting you to wake up and pay attention.

Establishing your Inner Sanctuary can be an individual practice, as it is in this chapter, or part of the beginning steps of a longer Yoga Nidra practice. It can be the same place or different each time. You simply need to close your eyes and visualize a place that makes you feel alive, happy, connected, and/or at peace by tapping into your senses. This can be an imaginary or a real place at an imagined or real time. You get to choose all the details of your Inner Sanctuary. It's your paradise. It's like a 10-minute time-share in your favorite place in the world along with the power to teleport there.

To establish your Inner Sanctuary, first consider what you might need in your life right now, similar to creating your Sankalpa. If you feel you need more nurturing, for example, remember or imagine a time when you felt cared for and all your needs were met. Otherwise, simply remember or imagine a time and place where you felt alive, happy, connected, and/or at peace. Then fill in the details or create them by drilling down on each of your senses. First, you'll imagine or remember the sights and sounds of your sanctuary. Then imagine or remember how it smells or tastes unique to this scene. Next, how does it feel? You may even include emotions, mind-set, and sense of spirit, though these aren't senses per se.

You'll be surprised at how effective this experience of visualizing your Inner Sanctuary is in calming you and making you feel completely alive. Visualizing your Inner Sanctuary is so simple, yet there are some very sophisticated things happening behind the scenes in your brain and body. Most important, this practice helps create a great foundation for your Yoga Nidra practice and acts as a home base you can return to at will for a quick reminder of what it feels like to experience your True Self.

What This Practice Does for You

The Inner Sanctuary practice, as well as Yoga Nidra in general, leverages your human senses to practice Awareness and therefore experience your True Nature. In this way, Yoga Nidra trains you to learn to somehow celebrate the fact that you may have stepped in dog poo on your way to work, because what a great way to practice being present and aware! "I'm simply welcoming, recognizing, and witnessing . . . dog poo. . . . It's neither good nor bad. . . . It's just information." Now that's some conscious shit!

Yoga Nidra is very safe to practice, but sometimes on our pathway to wholeness, we may become aware of difficult things to process, such as challenging emotions. In these instances, it is the part of you that is whole shedding the layers that keep you from experiencing your True Nature. No matter what arises for you, you can return to the safe haven of your Inner Sanctuary as needed. Remember, in Yoga Nidra, your job isn't to try to heal; it's only to practice Awareness. When you experience your True Self as Awareness, healing happens automatically. Nonetheless, you get to control how you practice Awareness, and visualizing your Inner Sanctuary is an excellent way to do that.

Some people dismiss the practice of visualizing as fantasizing or fetishizing something that isn't real. But, in fact, doing a visualization like establishing your Inner Sanctuary actually helps you create your reality. To borrow a line from *The Matrix*, "Real is simply electrical signals interpreted by your brain." Neuroscientists assert that our brains are not mirrors of reality but rather mere interpreters of it. Each person's brain is constantly bombarded by massive volumes of information every second of the day, even during sleep. Every brain attempts to interpret, sort, and organize all that information based on that person's previous experience. Each person's brain calls that interpretation of information "reality." Yet, given that each person has had invariably massively different experiences in life and therefore will always interpret information differently in both subtle and extreme ways, how could one person's reality possibly compare to another's? Nonetheless, we point to something we all call "reality" as if it were a monolithic object we can all agree on, when reality is actually subject to the interpretation of each person who is experiencing it.

With that said, we all know that our brains are poor interpreters of reality. Why else do your palms sweat during an intense movie even though you know it's not real? Whether seeing something in real life, watching it on a screen, or visualizing it in your head, your brain releases all the same chemicals into your body—chemicals like adrenaline, cortisol, and oxytocin. So, if what we call reality is what we can sense, and you can turn on your senses merely by thinking and imagining them, then quite veritably you can create your reality and fill your system with all the feel-good brain chemicals.

Visualizing your Inner Sanctuary can actually be more effective at making you feel at peace than if you were physically in a sanctuary. Think about this: A person could be sitting on one of the most beautiful beaches in the world, yet they may be lost in thought, worrying over something like money, oblivious to their senses and therefore the beach. Meanwhile, someone else is lying on their yoga mat practicing Yoga Nidra, thousands of miles from the ocean, experiencing the beach paradise.

This Inner Sanctuary titillates the practitioner's senses as they visualize the soft rays of the evening sun shimmer against the blue-green ocean, the fresh smell of the salt air filling their lungs, the soft sound of the gentle waves, the sweet taste of coconut water, and the warm, calm feeling in their heart, sensing the connectedness of all things. Between the stressed-out person sitting in the sand who is numb to the experience and the person who is completely connected to the experience in body, mind, and spirit, though thousands of miles away, tell me, which one is experiencing the beach?

I host yoga retreats around the world, and once, I was telling a friend about the mind-blowing sunsets during a retreat in southern Spain. He started belittling the sunsets in his hometown. Having never been to Spain, he then asked, "Do you think I'd like Spain?" to which I responded, "If you can't appreciate the sunset at home, you won't appreciate it in Spain." Whether you are on a retreat in Spain or in your own backyard, learning to visualize your Inner Sanctuary will allow you to access your peace and joy, even helping you recognize them in whatever's right in front of you.

5-MINUTE MEDITATION SCRIPT

This Yoga Nidra practice establishes your Inner Sanctuary. Practice simply welcoming, recognizing, and witnessing whatever arises.

Get comfortable. Close your eyes and release any tension with a few sighs.

Sense your entire body lying on the floor. Feel the upper half of your body as sensation. Feel only your lower half. Now feel both simultaneously. Feel your entire body.

Visualize your Inner Sanctuary—a place, real or imaginary, where you feel alive, happy, connected, and/or at peace.

First, notice what you see—shapes, colors, and textures. Pause for a moment as you absorb into your being what you see.

Now notice the smells in your sanctuary. Breathe in, and for a moment, simply allow this scent to fill up your entire being.

What do you hear in your sanctuary? Pick out two or three different sounds. For a moment, allow the sounds of your sanctuary to open up your entire being.

Now what do you taste in your sanctuary? Allow this taste to consume your entire being with peace, joy, and love.

What do you feel beneath your feet or at your fingertips? Give yourself over to the sensation of your skin.

What emotion do you feel while in your sanctuary? Is it a feeling of happiness, love, sensuality, connectedness, peace, calm . . . ? Allow that emotion to fill your entire being. For a moment, simply rest in this emotion.

Notice how your entire being feels while in your sanctuary. You can return to your sanctuary whenever you wish to be your best in life.

Now return your Awareness to your body lying on the floor. Practicing deep Awareness through Yoga Nidra and developing your Inner Sanctuary allows you to move throughout your life with a sustained sense of peace, love, and joy.

When you hear me count down from five (or ring the bell) that will signal the end of the Yoga Nidra practice.

5, 4, 3, 2, 1 (or ring the bell).

Yoga Nidra is over.

Get Started

Record either the short or long meditation (or both) in this chapter. As mentioned, developing your Inner Sanctuary can be a complete Yoga Nidra Practice in and of itself as well as the perfect foundation for a longer Yoga Nidra practice. It can also be a supplementary practice that you do outside of Yoga Nidra whenever you feel the need to visit your sanctuary. Again, it's like having the power to teleport to your own personal paradise whenever you wish, and who doesn't thrive in paradise? You're at your best when you feel relaxed, alive, and loving, which is what you'll feel in your Inner Sanctuary. You may choose to visualize your sanctuary as you go to sleep or as a midday pick-me-up or anytime you want to simply feel amazing.

Since our Inner Sanctuary leverages our senses to practice Awareness and experience our True Nature, I suggest making it a regular practice to delight in your senses. Experience the world the way a painter, poet, or photographer does. Wake up from being anesthetized by ordinary or numbed by normal, and start noticing the world's vivid colors and contrasts, ironies, and synchronicities. Begin noticing every flavor, smell, and touch.

Before developing your Inner Sanctuary in a Yoga Nidra practice, go on a sensory safari around your house. Take a walk from room to room and practice turning on your senses. Your housemates will think you're crazy for stroking the towels like they were an infant's tender head, rolling around on the wood floors with reckless abandon, and eating a square of dark chocolate like it were your last meal on earth. When they look at you like you've completely lost your sanity, simply inform them that it's they who are crazy for not noticing the ecstasy of sensation that is all around them, constantly begging them to pay attention. (After, you might need to find new housemates.)

Once you've tuned in to your senses, it's time to practice developing your Inner Sanctuary in a Yoga Nidra session. Set yourself up similar to any other Yoga Nidra practice. Minimize your distractions by establishing the right time and place to practice. Put your phone in airplane mode, close the door, hang your "Do Not Disturb" sign if you use one, and let the people you live with (assuming they still live with you) know that you'll be unavailable for a while. Arrange yourself on the floor with your yoga mat and place folded blankets on top with a roll or cushion under your knees and a folded blanket behind your head. Have your Yoga Nidra journal close by. Play back either the short or the long meditation from this chapter and guide yourself through your Inner Sanctuary. If distractions arise, simply witness them without any opinions.

If you'd like to practice your Inner Sanctuary outside of your Yoga Nidra practice, simply relax, close your eyes, take a few breaths, and begin the visualization process described in the scripts.

Reflect on Your Practice

As your Yoga Nidra practice concludes, give yourself a moment to come back into the feeling of your body. While still lying on the floor, give yourself a few deep breaths, remember what time of day it is, and gently open your eyes. When you're ready, roll over to one side and rest there for a few moments. Then sit up and give yourself a few more deep breaths. Notice if the feeling of your Inner Sanctuary lingers.

As you reflect on your practice, try to remember what happened during the practice. In your Yoga Nidra journal, spend a moment writing down your immediate responses to the practice. Though you are trying to see the world like a poet, you don't have to write about your experience like one. I encourage you to write freely without edits and simply get the words out. Just do a word dump onto the page. You can also respond to some or all of these questions in your journal:

⌀ What were you most aware of during this Yoga Nidra practice?

⌀ Did you stay awake, or did you fall asleep? Did you find yourself drifting between waking and dreaming?

⌀ What was your Inner Sanctuary like? Describe the details of your senses.

⌀ Was your Inner Sanctuary difficult to find or maintain?

⌀ How real did your Inner Sanctuary feel?

⌀ Did anything arise in your Awareness that you weren't
expecting? Were you able to return to your Inner Sanctuary?

If you found it difficult to find your Inner Sanctuary, don't worry.
This is a practice like everything else, and it will come in time.
Feel free to borrow another person's idea of paradise if necessary.
Sometimes, I visualize myself in Rivendell from *Lord of the Rings*,
simply because when I saw the movie I felt like Rivendell was a
place where I could be very comfortable.

It can be helpful to remember a time in your life when you felt
genuinely happy or when you laughed so hard that tears streamed
down your cheeks. These times and places could be your Inner
Sanctuary. Keep in mind, too, that your paradise could be something as simple as soaking in the bath with a good book; it doesn't
have to be grandiose. Again, in Yoga Nidra, nothing is supposed to
happen or not happen. Whatever happens does. Your only job is to
invite, acknowledge, and observe whatever arises in your field of
awareness. I encourage you to use your Inner Sanctuary as often
as possible. It's a simple practice with massive benefits.

Full Meditation Script

*Welcome to Yoga Nidra. Begin by lying down and getting as comfort-
able as possible. Close your eyes and release any unconscious tension by
giving yourself a few deep breaths in through the nose and out through
the mouth with deep sighs.*

*Sense your entire body lying on the floor. Feel your body as informa-
tion. Feel your head. Feel your arms. Feel yourself breathe. Feel your
back. Now feel your pelvis. Feel your legs from hips to knees, from knees
to lower legs, to ankles, feet, and toes.*

*Now feel only your upper half again as sensation. Feel only your
lower half. Upper half. Now feel both simultaneously. Feel your
entire body.*

What are you aware of in this moment? You may notice that as sensations are changing, they reveal a constant Awareness. Be the constant Awareness experiencing itself as a body lying on the floor. You are Awareness experiencing itself as the sensation of a body lying on the floor.

Now begin to visualize a place that for you is a sanctuary. This could be an actual or imaginary place and time. Choose a place where you can feel most alive, happy, connected, loving, or at peace. You get to decide all of the details as you visualize your sanctuary. You may change your sanctuary every time you practice Yoga Nidra.

Once you've chosen your sanctuary, notice the details using your senses.

Choose three or four things you see in your sanctuary, including shapes, colors, and textures. Rest for a moment as you see these objects. If you're inside, what do the walls, floor, and ceiling look like? If you're outside, what do the sky, clouds, or stars look like? Pause for a moment as you absorb into your being everything you see.

Switch your senses now and notice how it smells in your sanctuary. As you naturally breathe in, allow the scent of your sanctuary to fill up your entire being. Pause for a moment and simply be present to whatever you smell in your sanctuary.

Now what sounds do you hear in your sanctuary? Pick out two or three different sounds and notice whether they are loud or soft, close or far away. Do you hear music, or is there quiet? Allow the sounds of your sanctuary to open up your entire being and dance through you.

What do you taste in your sanctuary? Where do you taste this on your tongue? As you taste, how do you also smell this taste? Allow this taste to fill up your entire being with peace and happiness.

Now what does your skin feel in your sanctuary? What temperature is it? What do you feel beneath your feet or at your fingertips? Give yourself a minute to give yourself over to the sensation of your skin.

What emotion do you feel while in your sanctuary? Notice where in your body you feel that emotion. Is it a feeling of happiness, love, sensuality, or calm? Allow that emotion to fill your entire being. For a moment, simply experience this emotion.

Now notice how your entire being feels while in your sanctuary. This feeling is operating under the surface at all times, whether or not you're aware of it. You can return to this feeling whenever you wish to help you be your best in life.

In this moment, return your Awareness to the feeling of your body lying on the floor. Feel your hands, feet, and belly. Remember that you're practicing Yoga Nidra, what time of day it is, and everything you sense in this moment.

When you hear me count down from five (or ring the bell), that will signal the end of the Yoga Nidra practice. Practicing deep Awareness through Yoga Nidra and developing your Inner Sanctuary allow you to move throughout your life with a sustained sense of peace, love, and joy. You'll share this feeling with everyone around you merely by being in their presence.

5, 4, 3, 2, 1 (or ring the bell).
Yoga Nidra is over.

CHAPTER FOUR

STEP 3:
SCAN THE BODY

How to Do a Body Scan

Yoga Nidra is simply coming to know yourself as Awareness, and physical sensation is perhaps the easiest sensation to be aware of. During the body scan, while lying still, you will tap into how each part of your body feels, simply remaining aware of sensations as your attention moves from body part to body part. The body scan is perhaps the simplest way to practice Awareness because the senses provide you with constant information and are always inviting you to be present. As you'll experience while doing the meditations in this chapter, your entire Yoga Nidra practice could mostly consist of a body scan.

Some body scans start at the toes and slowly work upward, and others do the opposite. I prefer starting at the mouth and finishing at the feet. While there's no one correct way to do a body scan, I find it useful to emphasize the parts of the body that are particularly sensitive, such as the lips, hands, toes, and pelvis. For this reason, I usually start with the mouth, move on to other parts of the head, down the body, and then spend more time on the hands, pelvis, and feet. I may move my Awareness quickly through body parts like upper and lower arms and legs, but I'll usually spend the majority of time bringing my Awareness to the places where it gets more bang for its buck—in particularly sensitive areas.

Cultivating Awareness is not a linear thing, a step you take and then move on; it's actually circular, a practice you perform again and again, each time allowing you to experience a deeper and deeper layer of Awareness. That's why it's so helpful to listen to the same meditations several times. You'll notice this layered approach in the body scan scripts. You'll first open to a general and broad Awareness of your body before circling around to another body scan. When you revisit the body scan, you'll take the time to feel each part, especially the sensitive ones, with deepening levels of Awareness. And from there, you'll use what I call your Both/And nature, the product of moving from attention to Awareness.

What's the difference between attention and Awareness? Attention is what you're aware of in the moment, and Awareness is what is doing the observation. To see what I mean, toggle your attention by feeling the right hand, then left, then right, left, then both simultaneously. When you sense both hands at the same time, you get Both/And nature. Experiencing your Both/And nature is feeling yourself as two seemingly different things simultaneously in a way that expands your identity into Awareness itself. Suddenly you're neither yin nor yang; you're yin-yang. Then, from this more whole Awareness, you continue along the body scan and experience the other, less-sensitive parts of your body with deeper Awareness.

What This Practice Does for You

As you're learning, Yoga Nidra helps you disidentify from anything that isn't your True Self. In yogic philosophy, the body is one of the layers (the Annamaya kosha) that people identify with most often. The body, nonetheless, with all its senses, is one of the best tools you have to come to know your True Nature.

This chapter's body scan practice encourages you to distinguish between identifying with your body and simply being aware of it. Relaxed Awareness is the natural behavior of your True Self, and one of the most useful things a body scan does is systematically relax your body. The more you connect to Awareness, the more at ease you'll be.

A body and a mind that doesn't rest will eventually break down. Better rest equals a person who's more able to do all they need to do in a day. Pair that with your Both/And nature, and you have something of a superpower. One way to feel your Both/And nature is with the yin-yang marriage of consciousness and body—inhabiting your body and performing from that Awareness. This leads to an even greater Awareness and even greater ease moving through the world from that Awareness. Ultimately, it's the difference between merely doing an action to being it. This is embodied Awareness.

The body scan is also an excellent way to get grounded if you tend to disassociate from your body (that is, if you tend to live in your head or feel separate from your body when you meditate). When I first began practicing Yoga Nidra, I understood on an intellectual level that my True Nature was larger than my body, that it was Awareness itself. However, I felt as though I needed to transcend my body to experience something higher. But after practicing Yoga Nidra for a few years, I came to understand that Yoga Nidra is a non-dualist philosophy, a Both/And approach to knowing Self and the Universe. You can't find your way to enlightenment by ignoring your body—in fact, you're missing out on perhaps the greatest tool you possess toward spiritual awakening.

5-MINUTE MEDITATION SCRIPT

As you begin your Yoga Nidra practice, lie down and make yourself as comfortable as possible. Sigh through your mouth. Noticing all of your senses, invite, acknowledge, and observe anything in your Awareness.

Feel your entire body on the floor. Now feel the sensation of your mouth. Feel your lips, teeth, and tongue. Invite, acknowledge, and observe your mouth as sensation. There's nothing to do about it but simply witness your mouth as sensation.

Bring your attention to the sensation of your eyes. Now your ears. Feel your entire face: forehead, eyebrows, eyes, cheekbones, nose, lips, chin, and jaw. Feel all your facial pores open as if you've just washed with a warm washcloth.

Now feel the crown and back of the head. Feel your entire face. Now feel both your face and scalp simultaneously. Feel your entire head.

While what you are aware of changes, Awareness remains constant, revealing your Awareness by what you are aware of. Be Awareness, experiencing itself as sensation.

As Awareness, feel the sensation of your neck and throat. Feel your right arm: shoulder, upper arm, elbow, forearm, wrist, and hand. Feel your left arm: shoulder, upper arm, elbow, forearm, wrist, and hand. Now feel both arms simultaneously.

Feel your chest and belly. Feel your back. Now feel your entire trunk, front and back.

Feel the sensation of your pelvis. Feel your legs: hips, thighs, knees, lower legs, and feet. Feel heels, tops of the feet, soles, and toes.

Now feel the entire left side of your body. Feel the right side of your body. Left side. Right side. Now feel the entire body. Notice again that what you are aware of changes, but Awareness stays constant. The sensations change and reveal constant Awareness. Be unchanging Awareness.

> When you hear me count down from five (or ring the bell), that will signal the end of the Yoga Nidra practice. To close, feel your hands and feet. When we finish, you'll move through your day feeling alive, embodied, and energized.
>
> 5, 4, 3, 2, 1 (or ring the bell).
>
> Yoga Nidra is over.

Get Started

Record either the short or long meditation (or both) in this chapter. Before you settle in for Yoga Nidra, take time to connect with and appreciate your body. As suggested in chapter 2, you can connect to your senses by walking around the house and feeling, smelling, and looking at all the different sensory delights. Pay extra-close attention to the sensation of your body. Notice pressure, texture, temperature, and so on. Feel your body as it moves. You may even want to rub your body with lotion or coconut oil or get a massage.

You could also try a few gentle yoga poses to help you connect to your body. Yoga poses are the perfect prep for a Yoga Nidra practice in general—but especially one that focuses on a body scan. Grounding poses such as Paschimottanasana (Seated Forward Fold Pose), Supta Kapotasana (Supine Figure Four Pose), and Jathara Parivartanasana (Supine Abdominal Twist) are good choices. (See the resources section on page 136 for a link to view these poses.) Yoga poses have a nice way of making you aware of and getting comfortable with your limitations. Always err on the side of too easy rather than too difficult. Remember that you're not trying to get a workout but rather connect to your body. While doing poses, maintain a deep, slow breath.

Once you feel more connected to your body, set up your Yoga Nidra nest as described previously and prepare to practice. Remember to put your phone in airplane mode, minimize other distractions, and have your Yoga Nidra journal handy.

If you have a difficult time connecting to your body, you may wish to place something relatively heavy, say around five pounds or less, on your chest, belly, pelvis, or thighs while you practice. Yoga gear outfitters sell sandbags for this purpose. They are long, heavy sacks with handles that you can place on your body to help you feel grounded. You can improvise and make your own by filling up a plastic ziplock bag with sand, flour, sugar, or small rocks and wrapping it in a towel. Another idea for grounding during your practice is to place two unopened cans of soup in your hands. Lying under a heavy quilt can also help you stay grounded and at ease if it doesn't make you too hot.

Reflect on Your Practice

As your Yoga Nidra practice concludes, give yourself a moment to come back into the feeling of the present moment. Notice how your body feels after doing a practice that focused so much on your body. Sometimes, after connecting to my Awareness with an extended body scan, I feel like my body is a heavy glove wrapped around my underlying essence, which is light and luminous.

Give yourself a few deep breaths, and open your eyes. Begin to move your fingers and toes very consciously and slowly. When you're ready, roll onto your side and rest in that position for a moment, and then sit up. Give yourself a few more deep breaths. Notice how your body feels.

As you reflect on your practice, describe to yourself what happened. In your Yoga Nidra journal, spend a moment writing down your immediate responses to the practice. As always, I encourage you to write freely without edits. You can also respond to some or all of these questions in your journal:

⌀ What were you most aware of during this Yoga
   Nidra practice?

⊘ Did you find that the body scan helped you become relaxed?

⊘ Did you stay awake, or did you fall asleep? Did you find yourself drifting between waking and dreaming?

⊘ What came into your Awareness as you focused on your body?

⊘ Was it difficult to maintain a focus on your body, or did you tend to focus on other parts of your being like thoughts, energy, or emotion?

⊘ Did anything spontaneously arise in your Awareness that you weren't expecting?

⊘ How does your body feel after the body scan?

If you found it difficult to connect to your body, don't worry. Just like all the other elements in this book, it's a practice, and it will come in time. Some people connect more readily to thoughts and emotions, other people to body, and others to energy. Everyone is different. This 10-step method familiarizes you with all the tools so you can choose the ones that work best for you.

Often, doing a body scan is very useful for a quick check-in and instant grounding. Before starting a teacher training, class, or lecture, I'll often invite my students to check in to their bodies by leading them through a one-minute body scan. It's incredible how quickly the energy in the room goes from frenetic and volatile to calm and controlled.

Occasionally I may have an expansive experience while practicing Yoga Nidra, where I feel my Awareness floating above my body or my mind soaring through space. When this happens, I do a brief body scan to reground me. It usually helps me experience the embodied Awareness feeling I mentioned earlier, and afterward,

I feel like I could run an Ironman Triathlon. This is how the professional athletes and performers say they've felt when they have used Yoga Nidra to help them perform.

Full Meditation Script

Welcome to Yoga Nidra. Lie down and make yourself as comfortable as possible. Release any tension with a few breaths in through your nose and out through your mouth with a sigh.

Start by noticing your senses. Notice the sounds, the smells, and the feeling of your body. You may be aware of thoughts or emotions. Simply invite, acknowledge, and observe anything and everything that enters your Awareness.

In this moment, open your attention to the sensation of your body lying on the floor. Notice your entire body, no single part in particular but your entire body. Now bring all of your attention to the sensation of your mouth. Feel your lips, your teeth, and your tongue. Now feel your entire mouth as sensation. Invite, acknowledge, and observe your entire mouth as sensation. There's nothing to do about it but simply witness your mouth as sensation.

Bring your attention to the sensation of your eyes. Feel your eyeballs in their sockets. Now ears. Feel your ears as sensation. Notice the feeling of your earlobes, the curves of your ears, and even sense the ear canals that recede into your skull.

Feel the sensation of your entire face. Feel your forehead, your eyebrows, your eyes, cheekbones, nose, lips, chin, and jaw. Adopt the feeling of all of the pores in your face opening as if you've just washed your face with a warm washcloth.

Bring your attention to the crown of your head. Now feel the back of your head resting on the floor or cushion. Now feel your entire face. In this moment, feel both your face and your scalp simultaneously. Feel your entire head.

While what you are aware of changes, Awareness remains constant. You reveal your Awareness by what you are aware of. Changing sensations illuminate your constant Awareness. Be Awareness itself, experiencing itself as the sensation.

As Awareness itself, feel the sensation of your neck and throat. Bring your attention to the sensation of your left arm, your entire left arm. Now feel your left shoulder, your upper arm, elbow, forearm, wrist, and hand. Feel the sensation of only your left thumb, first finger, middle finger, fourth finger, and little finger. Now feel your entire left arm.

Bring your attention to the sensation of your entire right arm. Feel your right shoulder, upper arm, elbow, forearm, wrist, and hand. Feel only your right thumb, first finger, middle finger, fourth finger, and little finger. Now feel your entire right arm. Now feel both arms simultaneously.

Bring your attention to the feeling of your chest. Notice the movement of your breath. Perhaps you can even sense the gentle beating of your heart. Feel your belly. Now feel your shoulder blades, your spine, and lower back. Feel your entire back, feel your entire front, back, front. Now feel your entire trunk, your chest, belly, and back.

Feel the sensation of your pelvis. Trace the sensation of your left leg beginning with your left hip, thigh, knee, lower leg, and foot. Feel your left heel, top of the foot, sole, and toes. Now feel the sensation of your right leg beginning with your right hip, thigh, knee, lower leg, and foot. Feel your right heel, top of the foot, sole, and toes.

Feel the sensation of the entire left side of your body, head to toe. Now feel the sensation of the entire right side of your body, head to toe. Left side. Right side. Now feel the sensation of your entire body at the same time. Feel your entire body.

Notice again that what you are aware of changes, but Awareness stays constant. The sensations change and reveal a constant Awareness. Be the unchanging Awareness.

Bring your attention back to the feeling of your breath moving in and out of your chest. Feel the palms of your hands and the soles of your feet. When you hear me count down from five (or ring the bell), that will signal the end of the Yoga Nidra practice, and you'll move throughout your day feeling alive, embodied, and energized.

5, 4, 3, 2, 1 (or ring the bell).

Yoga Nidra is over.

CHAPTER FIVE

STEP 4: FOLLOW THE BREATH

How to Tune In to Your Breath

The breath serves as an excellent anchor for meditation. Your body is constantly breathing, and with only two components—inhalations and exhalations—breathing is usually easy to focus on. It's just an exhale followed by an inhale. In a universe of constant change, focusing on the continuity of your breath is similar to finding solace in the sound of waves gently crashing on the beach. Within the movement of your breath, you also find stillness. This is another paradox that helps us understand the part of us that is connected to everything else. It's a way of experiencing our Both/And nature.

There are a few simple breathing techniques that can help you build your Awareness and prepare you to practice Yoga Nidra.

So far, I've only discussed giving yourself a few deep breaths. Now I'd like to share with you my go-to breathing practice before we move on. It is called Ujjayi (pronounced *oo-jie-ee*) Breath, sometimes called Whisper Breath or Victorious Breath.

Ujjayi Breath is performed by taking deep breaths in and out of your nose, with your inhalation lasting 4 to 6 seconds and your exhalations lasting 5 to 7 seconds. One of the ways to elongate your breath is to very slightly constrict the muscles in the back of your throat the way you would when you whisper. As you practice this technique, you can feel and hear the "whisper" with every breath. Keep your jaw relaxed during this practice to avoid becoming tense.

If this breathing style makes you feel dizzy or as if you can't catch your breath, it could be the product of constricting your throat too much. Lessen the tension in your throat muscles or stop constricting them altogether and just focus on deep breaths. Dizziness could result from emphasizing your inhale over your exhale, so try elongating your exhale a bit more to see if that helps.

When I first started yoga, I practiced in front of a mirror. I would often catch glimpses of myself looking wild and bug-eyed and found that while trying to maintain the pose and Ujjayi Breath, I could never get enough air. It turned out I was constricting my throat too much and wasn't allowing myself to breathe deeply enough. Ujjayi Breath, which should have been facilitating my practice, was actually hindering it. As soon as I pumped the brakes a little on my throat constriction, I found Ujjayi Breath to be much more enjoyable and consequently very helpful to my yoga practice.

What This Practice Does for You

Connecting to your breath is an excellent way to build Awareness. It's also the easiest way to access the part of you that is subtler than your body but that you can still feel. In Yoga Nidra, this part of you is called the subtle body, or the Pranamaya kosha. It is the part of you that feels energy, emotions like anger and happiness, and feelings like heaviness or lightness.

Prana is the Sanskrit word for "energy." It is thought to make everything in the Universe move—from atoms and galaxies to thoughts and emotions. Even if you're not sure what they are, you've probably heard of chakras. They are energy centers within the subtle body that you can think of like subway stations for prana. The goal of movement, breathing, and mindfulness in yoga is to keep prana flowing through your chakras to avoid stagnation. Connecting with your breath helps keep the energy flowing from hub to hub.

We are all familiar with the effects of prana, though we probably give it another name like energy, vibes, or juju. For instance, have you ever stared at the back of someone ahead of you when suddenly they turn around to see whose eyes were boring into their head? Weird, right? Or have you ever been thinking about someone and they happen to call you right then? Most of us have probably experienced such scenarios; they're the product of prana.

You have much more control over the energy within and around you than you may think. Learning to control and focus on your breath helps you understand and control how energy moves in your life and can actually help you energize those parts of your life that need some vitality, even parts like your finances, romance, or emotions. By focusing on your breath in Yoga Nidra, you can truly breathe energy into all parts of your life.

Thinking about your breath is the perfect way to begin to connect to and direct energy. Try this simple energy experiment: Close your eyes and simply feel both of your hands. Then begin to think of your favorite color, and with each inhale, visualize your breath becoming that color and moving from your nose through your right arm and all the way down into your right hand. With each exhale, picture your colored breath moving back up your arm and out through your nose. Continue this for a few minutes and then notice if one hand feels different from the other. If so, this is prana. If you don't feel anything, it doesn't mean you did anything wrong. Maybe you connect with prana in different ways. Maybe you express prana in your ability to analyze or conceptualize things. If you're more analytical, try the same experiment but simply focus on the center of your palm and commit to steady breaths.

Remember, each person connects to Awareness in different ways. Some people connect very easily through the body and senses, while others might connect more through energy, breath, and emotions. In Yoga Nidra, we explore all the layers that we might identify with as the method of expanding into Awareness.

5-MINUTE MEDITATION SCRIPT

To begin this Yoga Nidra practice, start by breathing in through your nose and sighing out through your mouth a few times. Simply invite, acknowledge, and observe anything in your Awareness. Repeat your Sankalpa in your head if you have one.

Without controlling it, simply notice your breathing. Feel yourself breathe into your face, entire head, arms, chest, belly, back, pelvis, legs, and feet. Where do you feel energy in your body in this moment? Simply invite, acknowledge, and observe energy manifesting in this moment.

Feel the floor of your pelvis, and imagine a bright red glow. Picture your favorite spot on earth. Remember when you felt at home. Notice your energy.

Feel your lower abdomen, and imagine a bright orange glow. Picture your favorite body of water. Remember a time when you could go with the flow of the events of your life. Notice your energy.

Feel your belly, and imagine a bright yellow glow. Remember feeling the sun on your skin. Remember feeling powerful. Notice your energy.

Feel your heart, and imagine a bright green glow. Remember your favorite green space. What is something you love without reservation? Notice your energy.

Feel the center of your throat, and imagine a bright sky-blue glow. Picture looking up into the clouds, lost in the blue sky. Remember speaking truth and trust. Notice your energy.

Feel the center of your forehead, and imagine an indigo glow. Picture floating in the atmosphere. Remember a time of deep inner knowing. Notice your energy.

Finally, feel your crown, and imagine a violet glow. Picture yourself floating in space. Remember feeling connected to everything. Notice your energy.

Feel your body on the floor. Because you practiced feeling the energy, you'll be able to powerfully direct the flow of energy in your life to manifest where you need it. When you hear me count down from five (or ring the bell), that will signal the end of the Yoga Nidra practice.

5, 4, 3, 2, 1 (or ring the bell).

Yoga Nidra is over.

Get Started

Record either the short or long meditation (or both) in this chapter. As always, choose a time and a place to practice Yoga Nidra when you stand the best chance of not being disturbed. Put your phone in airplane mode, place your sign on the door if you use one, and keep your Yoga Nidra journal close by. Have your cushions, blankets, and pillows available, but this time, place them off the mat so that you can do a few yoga poses and practice Ujjayi Breath before you start Yoga Nidra practice.

Doing the few gentle yoga poses described next in tandem with Ujjayi Breath is an excellent way to focus your energy and Awareness as you prepare for Yoga Nidra. Negotiate the intensity of every pose to stay within your comfortable limits.

JANU SHIRSHASANA (HEAD-TO-KNEE POSE). Sit on the floor, or on a cushion if you have tight legs, resting your right foot on the inside of your left leg. Reach for your left toes or shin until you feel a comfortable stretch. Try to keep the stretch in the belly of the hamstrings (back of the thigh). Bend your knee if it's more comfortable. Use Ujjayi Breath and visualize your breath moving into your hamstrings. Hold this pose for 10 to 15 breaths on each side.

SUPTA KAPOTASANA (SUPINE FIGURE FOUR POSE). Lie on your back and cross your right leg over the left thigh. The left foot could stay on the floor if this is intense. Remember to relax your jaw and breathe slowly using Ujjayi Breath. Visualize your breath moving in and out of the place where you feel this stretch. Hold this pose for 10 to 15 breaths on each side with a little rest between sides.

SUPTA BADDHA KONASANA (SUPINE COBBLER'S POSE). While sitting on the mat, lie back over a cushion and with your feet together, open your knees, and rest each knee on a cushion. Place your hands on your belly and practice using Ujjayi Breath to bring energy down into your belly, pelvis, and legs. Hold this pose for 15 to 20 breaths.

After your poses, lie or sit on your mat and do one or both of these exercises:

UJJAYI BREATH. Controlling your breath is a very effective way to help you calm your nervous system to enter into the state of relaxed Awareness we are searching for in Yoga Nidra. Using Ujjayi Breath, allow all of your attention to merely focus on the sound and feeling of your breath. Maintain this for a few minutes.

COUNTDOWN MEDITATION. Set a timer for 5 minutes, and using Ujjayi Breath or not, start with the number 30 and begin to count your breaths down to zero. As you exhale, think the number, "30," inhale and think, "29," exhale, "28," etc. If you lose your count, simply start over. If you get to zero, start over. Whether you start 100 times or get to zero several times, there is no goal other than to remain focused on your breath.

After you've practiced your poses and have done your breathing practice, arrange yourself to be comfortable in your Yoga Nidra practice, abandon your Ujjayi Breath, and play back your recording.

Reflect on Your Practice

As your Yoga Nidra practice concludes, take a moment to notice how energy feels in your body. Remember that energy can feel all kinds of ways in your body—electric, dull, light, heavy, cool, etc. Energy might also evoke colors, thoughts, images (like quick snapshots in your mind), or emotions.

After you've had a moment to feel this experience, roll over onto your side and rest in this position for a moment, then sit up. In your Yoga Nidra journal, give yourself a moment to write down your immediate responses to the practice and describe to yourself what you experienced. Remember, the idea is just to do a word dump onto the page. You can also respond to some or all of these questions in your journal:

- What were you most aware of during this Yoga Nidra practice?

- How did energy manifest to you in your practice?

- Did you stay awake, or did you fall asleep? Did you find yourself drifting between waking and dreaming?

- What came into your Awareness as you focused on your energy?

- What, if any, were the insights you came to as you practiced?

- Was it difficult to maintain a focus on your energy, or did you tend to focus on other parts of your being like thoughts or emotions?

- During the practice, did anything spontaneously arise in your Awareness that you weren't expecting?

- How do you feel following this energy practice?

- What are the areas in your life that feel like they could use a little more energy?

If you found it difficult to connect to energy, you're not alone. Everybody has their own way of connecting. Some people just don't relate to the world in terms of energy. This might be you if you tend to be more analytical in your thinking. Remember that energy, or prana, is about movement, change, and form. You might experience prana through ideas, concepts, or analysis. It's important to begin to recognize all the ways prana moves in your life.

If you found that it was easy to connect to the feeling of prana, take a moment after this practice to picture energy flowing into the areas in your life that could use a little more vitality. Maybe you need to see some changes at work, in your love life, your finances, or whatever. As abstract as this seems, practice the Ujjayi Breath while visualizing the area of your life you would like to see receive more energy.

Remember that prana lies somewhere between thought and breath. Setting a Sankalpa is like blowing life into an idea and watching it come alive. Once you learn to master your prana, you'll find ways to set prana in motion toward the things you need and want. For this purpose, it's useful to repeat your Sankalpa often and direct prana toward what serves you. If you didn't have a Sankalpa the first time you did this energy practice, try setting one next time.

Full Meditation Script

Welcome to Yoga Nidra. Lie down and make yourself as comfortable as possible. Clear any excess energy by breathing in through the nose, holding your breath for just a second, and letting it go with a sigh. Do this a few times and then breathe naturally.

Notice your surroundings. Notice any thoughts and emotions you have at this moment. Practice welcoming, recognizing, and witnessing anything you're aware of in this moment, either internal or external. Repeat your Sankalpa in your head a few times if you have one.

Abandon any control of your breath and simply notice your breathing. Without changing your breath, feel as if you are breathing into your entire face. Now breathe into your entire head. Breathe into your arms. Chest and belly. Back. Pelvis. Legs. Feet.

Breathe into only the front side of your body. Feel as if your entire front side gets bigger with each breath. Now breathe into only the back side of your body and feel as if your entire back side gets bigger with each breath. Front side. Back side. Now breathe into your entire body. Your entire body is breathing.

Notice how you feel energy in this moment. Where in your body do you feel energy? How would you describe this energy? Is it sharp or dull? Is it moving or still? Are there colors connected to the way energy feels in your body? What are all the ways feeling energy in this moment affects you? Simply invite, acknowledge, and observe any way that energy manifests in this moment.

Bring your attention to the floor of your pelvis and notice the energy there. This is your first chakra. Imagine a bright red glow. Picture your favorite spot on earth, a garden, a trail, or a beach. Now remember a time when you felt at home. Notice how your energy feels in this moment.

Now bring your attention to your lower abdomen. This is your second chakra. Imagine a bright orange glow. Picture your favorite body of water. Remember a time when you were able to go with the flow of any events in your life. Notice how your energy feels in this moment.

Now bring your attention to your belly. This is your third chakra. Imagine a bright yellow glow. Picture a time when you enjoyed feeling the sun on your skin. Now remember feeling powerful in your life. Notice how your energy feels in this moment.

Bring your attention to your heart. This is your fourth chakra. Imagine a bright green glow. Remember your favorite green space, a forest, field, or garden. What is something you love without reservation? Notice how your energy feels in this moment.

Place your attention on the center of your throat. This is your fifth chakra. Imagine a bright sky-blue glow. Picture looking up into the clouds, lost in the blue sky. Remember a time when you felt that you spoke your truth, trusting that you would be heard. Notice how you feel in this moment.

Move your attention to the center of your forehead. This is your sixth chakra. Imagine an indigo glow, an iridescent blue-purple. Picture floating high in the atmosphere. Remember a time of deep inner knowing. Notice how your energy feels in this moment.

Finally, move your attention to the crown of your head. This is your seventh chakra. Imagine a violet glow reaching toward the heavens. Picture yourself floating in space without an up or down, right or left. Remember a time when you felt connected to all things. Notice how you feel in this moment.

Bring your attention to the feeling of energy through your entire body. You may even feel energy outside your body. While energy is constantly changing, it reveals that which is never changing: your Awareness. Be the unchanging Awareness.

Experience your body on the floor by feeling your hands and feet, chest and belly. When you hear me count down from five (or ring the bell), that will signal the end of the Yoga Nidra practice. Because you've practiced feeling the energy in your body, you'll be able to powerfully direct the flow of energy in your life to manifest where you need it.

5, 4, 3, 2, 1 (or ring the bell).

Yoga Nidra is over.

CHAPTER SIX

STEP 5: TURN TOWARD EMOTIONS

How to Listen to Your Emotions

Turning toward your emotions means witnessing them as an objective observer. This can help you learn to respond rather than react to your emotions in your day-to-day life. By this point in the 10-step method, you've become familiar with witnessing the sensations and energy of your body—including things like hot and cold, heavy and light, etc. Learning to witness the body and energy will help you witness your emotions with the same level of objectivity and perspective as you would to, say, the sensation in your hands.

There's a distinction here between feelings and emotions: Feelings refer to the experience of a sensation (felt sense), and emotions refer to qualities like happy and sad. Yoga Nidra teaches you to invite, acknowledge, and observe—not react to—emotions. A great response to almost any emotion is a big breath. When a big emotion arises, like anger, fright, or sadness, try first taking a big breath and welcoming the emotion with the phrase "Emotions are part of a normal human experience." I know—sounds über-obvious, but it's incredible how often emotions eclipse our perspective and suddenly the entire Universe exists only as that red-hot emotion burning in your gut. Even with a simple assurance that emotions are normal, you grant yourself a perspective that may help you respond rather than react.

Next, recognize the emotion. In addition to calling it what it is—an emotion—notice all the ways it affects you. Where do you feel that emotion in your body? How would you describe it to yourself? Does it evoke a feeling like pressure, heat, or spaciousness? Does it conjure thoughts, memories, or other emotions? Now practice merely witnessing the emotion without doing anything about it. Again, remind yourself that it's normal to have this emotion.

Often, an emotion is a call to action. So ask yourself: "What's this anger I feel in my heart asking me to do?" If you feel you need to respond to your emotion after observing it, you'll do so from a grounded place, well away from reaction.

I can tell you from experience that this practice of responding and not reacting to emotions is a lifetime practice. But learning to witness my emotions rather than immediately reacting to them has been a life changer for me. For example, when someone cuts me off in traffic, I'm learning to first feel the anger of the moment, take a deep breath, and then stay focused on what I need to do to be safe in the moment rather than yelling. Then, the next time similar emotions come around, I can see them for what they are rather than getting swept up in the same tide of reaction. That's not to say I don't ever get provoked to anger and occasionally use some of my favorite four-letter words—you know, those other than *hope*, *love*, and *nice*.

Through Yoga Nidra, you can gain perspective and awareness of emotions, whether they're pleasant or uncomfortable. Once, I heard a Sanskrit scholar recount the tale of a yoga guru who'd experienced enlightenment. He was surrounded by his students who said to their guru that it must be nice not to feel anger anymore. The guru responded to the students with, "Oh, anger! That's one of my favorite emotions!" He was teaching them that enlightenment doesn't mean being separate from emotions but rather learning to understand them as a pathway to understanding your True Self.

What This Practice Does for You

Your emotions belong to the next level of koshas: the Manomaya kosha. Because you feel them in your body and they are the product of prana (energy), emotions are the perfect blend of the previous two koshas, the body layer (Annamaya kosha) and the energy layer (Pranamaya kosha). One of my students was an incredible runner who used anger and heartache to fuel his runs. Instead of reacting to these emotions, he channeled that energy into movement.

It's easy to label some emotions like happiness as good and other emotions like anger as bad. You want to experience some emotions, but others you hope to avoid at all costs. You can even identify your entire existence with them, as if you were a Care Bear whose name denotes your most prominent emotion (hello, Grumpy Bear). But the truth is, anything you identify with other than your True Self is setting you up for an existential crisis. Emotions are perhaps one of the parts of your humanity that is the most volatile.

Have you ever been offended by someone offering you help and then had those feelings replaced by gratitude after you realized how much you benefitted from that help? Or have you ever felt criticized by someone's comment that really had nothing to do with you? Humans are constantly interpreting the events that happen (and don't happen) and labeling them good or bad, triggering an entire suite of emotions. But there is no absolute truth in emotions (beyond the fact that you're feeling them); there's only interpretation. Practices like Yoga Nidra reveal that emotions are merely a human experience and the product of how your mind interprets the events in your life.

Just as you might witness the sensation of your body with mild interest, so, too, can you learn to witness emotions with something like "Hmm. How interesting. There's sadness again." Responsiveness puts you in control of your emotions rather than feeling like your emotions control you. That doesn't mean you need to act like a robot and never feel emotions like sadness, for example. It's just the opposite. As someone who was afraid of emotions for many years, I know how drab life can be without them. Yoga Nidra was one of the most beautiful tools I discovered to switch my emotional radar back on by teaching me there is nothing to fear, that emotions are normal, and that I am much larger than whatever is coming up.

I remember the day my emotional radar turned back on. It was after a particularly deep Yoga Nidra practice where I felt myself at one with the Universe. I came home that night and for about four hours sat in a chair in my bathrobe and alternately cried my eyes out and laughed my eyes out, each cycle switching every 10 minutes or so. Since that moment, I have felt free to experience the full spectrum of emotions—from despair and sadness to ecstatic joy, each one reminding me that I'm truly aware and alive.

5-MINUTE MEDITATION SCRIPT

To begin this Yoga Nidra practice, start by breathing in through your nose and sighing out through your mouth a few times. Notice everything around you. Be curious about any emotion you feel in this moment.

Repeat your Sankalpa to yourself if you have one. Establish your Inner Sanctuary. At any time, you may return to this place.

Now feel your entire body. Mouth. Eyes. Ears. Nose. Crown. Back of head. Entire face. Scalp. Face. Scalp. Arms. Hands. Feel both hands simultaneously. Feel chest. Belly. Back. Pelvis. Legs. Feet.

What are you aware of in this moment? Be unchanging Awareness. Feel yourself as large. Now small. Large. Small. Now be both small and large.

What's something that makes you happy? Fill in the details of this happy scene by noticing your senses: the sights, sounds, smells, tastes, and sensations.

Where do you feel happiness in your body? What are all the ways you feel happiness? Invite, acknowledge, and observe happiness.

If it feels safe to do so, remember feeling disappointment. If not, remember boredom. Fill in the details of this scene by noticing your senses: the sights, sounds, smells, tastes, and sensations. Witness how this emotion feels in your body. Notice all the ways this emotion affects your being.

Let go of disappointment or boredom, and pick up happiness. Remember the scene of happiness. Release happiness and pick up disappointment or boredom. Happiness. Disappointment or boredom. Now feel both simultaneously. Feel the part of you that is large enough to feel both emotions.

Repeat in your mind, "Though I have emotions, I am larger than emotions. Each emotion is pointing me to Awareness."

Bring your attention back to your body, your Inner Sanctuary, and your Sankalpa if you had one. When you hear me count down from five (or ring the bell), that will signal the end of the Yoga Nidra practice. Because you've practiced Awareness through emotions today, you'll have the power to respond effectively to the emotions that visit you in your life.

5, 4, 3, 2, 1 (or ring the bell).

Yoga Nidra is over.

Get Started

Record either the short or long meditation (or both) in this chapter. Set a time and a place that will be best for you to practice. Make all your usual preparations to set up your Yoga Nidra nest. For this practice, you may want to have a box of tissues handy. Of course, there is no shortage of opportunities to practice Awareness through emotions, but here's a simple practice you can do to help train you to invite, acknowledge, and observe emotions.

Choose 5 to 10 photos that tend to make you feel happiness, excitement, or love. They could be photos of family, friends, pets, or places you really enjoy. Spend at least 60 seconds looking at each photo. As you look at the photo, notice the emotion that each photo evokes. Then close your eyes and ask yourself the following questions:

🖋 What emotion do I feel?

🖋 Where do I feel it in my body?

🖋 Does the emotion have a color? Which one?

🖋 What, if any, are the feelings this emotion evokes, like hot/cold, heavy/light, expanded/contracted, etc.?

🖋 Does this emotion evoke thoughts, memories, or images?

🖋 Are there any other ways this emotion manifests in my being?

Then, once you've answered those questions, practice simply witnessing that emotion. Don't hold on to or resist the emotion. Simply witness it. Repeat to yourself, "Though I have emotions, I'm bigger than emotions. Emotions will come and go, but each one is an opportunity to practice Awareness." Just like learning to take the time to truly savor food, so, too, can we learn to savor emotions. Go through this same process with each photo. Different photos of the same subject might evoke different emotions.

Since emotions are so closely related to your energy, it's useful to do breathing exercises prior to Yoga Nidra to prime your energy to facilitate emotions. While either sitting on a cushion with your legs crossed or lying down in your Yoga Nidra position, practice using Ujjayi Breath (see page 46) as you visualize your breath moving from your head to your toes as you inhale and from your toes all the way back up to your head as you exhale. The idea is to simply feel energy begin to move through your body. Emotions have a cycle and a flow. These breathing exercises simply clear the way through your energy channels so emotions can come and go and not get repressed or stuck. It's like cleaning out the straw before drinking through it but for energy.

While learning to invite, acknowledge, and observe emotions is a valuable practice, certain emotions can be very painful and traumatic. Establishing your Inner Sanctuary (see page 23) is a beneficial way to prepare to work with emotions, because if anything arises that you weren't expecting or that is too difficult to work with, you're welcome to bring yourself back to your sanctuary and allow your safe haven to help ground you.

With Awareness, you can learn to simply be with even the most difficult emotions, but be gentle with yourself, because this is a practice and you don't need to try to hold your deepest trauma right away. Instead, just develop your Awareness as it pertains to gentler emotions and allow the work of holding anything more difficult to happen naturally. Keep in mind that you're not trying to heal; healing just happens as the product of Awareness. While you may not have control of everything that pops into your Awareness, you can navigate your way through whatever arises by using tools like your Inner Sanctuary.

Reflect on Your Practice

As your Yoga Nidra practice concludes, take a moment to come back into the feeling of your body. If you have any lingering emotions, practice welcoming, recognizing, and witnessing them. You may wish to respond to those emotions with a few deep breaths or perhaps a few sighs through your mouth. Repeat the phrase you established in your Yoga Nidra practice, "Though I have emotions, I am larger than emotions. Each emotion is pointing me to Awareness." When you're ready, roll over onto your side and rest in that position for a moment, and then sit up. In your Yoga Nidra journal, spend a moment writing down your immediate responses to the practice without editing.

Remember that emotions are often a call to action. Your body is usually the best or first tool you can use to respond. Even if it seems unrelated to what you're experiencing at the moment, regularly move your body to help you process and express your emotions. Especially in the privacy of your Yoga Nidra space, perhaps you might try dancing to whatever arises. If whipping out a modern, interpretive number just isn't your thing, try doing some yoga poses, lifting weights, going on a walk or hike, or riding your bike. Also, taking a shower or bath and connecting to the sensations of your body is very helpful to begin processing emotions. Anything that connects you to your body is valuable. The American poet Wallace Stevens once wrote, "Perhaps the truth depends on a walk around the lake." If you have a lake nearby, try it.

It's extremely valuable to find a trusted friend with whom you can regularly express your emotions. Having someone to talk to about emotions is an essential part of learning to invite, acknowledge, and observe them (aka "hold them"). A good friend can also reflect your emotions back to you and offer clarity and insight. One of my clients often speaks enthusiastically about her "paid friend" (her therapist who helps her discern her emotions the way a good friend might).

Yoga Nidra has helped me manage many intense emotions. Years ago, while in a yoga class, I began to suffer a panic attack. I had just put my students in Savasana and was sitting on my mat looking serene on the outside, but on the inside, I felt like my heart was being stabbed with a hot knife. Unfortunately, at this time, I was having frequent panic attacks. The two yoga studios I'd built were bleeding money, and it was obvious they would soon take their last breaths. I was worried sick. I felt sad that all the time, money, and effort I had put into the studios would be lost. I felt guilty about all the students and teachers I'd be letting down when the studios closed. I felt angry that vital information about the location of one of my studios, which ultimately caused it to fail, had been withheld when I signed my lease.

I knew all the yoga tricks and visualizations that would help allay these emotions, but instead, I chose to greet them head-on by welcoming, recognizing, and witnessing them. I described to myself how they felt. I noticed that the sensation around my chest felt more like a breastplate of armor rather than a hot knife. Suddenly, my emotions were protecting me against the calamity and calling me to fight for whatever I could save. With this reframe, my emotions became fuel for action instead of pointless panic. That moment broke the momentum of my panic attacks, and while the next several months were not easy, the panic attacks stopped because I was willing to greet the pain rather than run from it.

Full Meditation Script

Welcome to Yoga Nidra. Lie down and make yourself as comfortable as possible. Begin by opening your Awareness to everything around you. Notice the sounds, the smells, and the temperature in the room. Bring your attention inside and notice if you're starting your practice with a particular emotion. Simply be curious about that emotion.

If you would like to use a Sankalpa in your practice, create your brief statement of truth that is positive, specific, and present, and repeat this a few times in your head.

Next, establish your Inner Sanctuary by remembering or imagining a place that you love to be, where you can be your best. Move through each of your senses as you evoke the feelings of your sanctuary. Remember that you may return to this place anytime you wish, especially if there are any emotions that arise that you don't want to work with in the moment.

At any time during this practice, you may return to your Inner Sanctuary.

Now feel your body lying on the floor, your entire body. Feel your mouth. Feel your eyes, ears, and nose. Feel the crown of your head. Now the back of your head. Feel your entire face. Now feel your entire scalp. Face. Scalp. Now feel your entire head at once. Feel your entire head.

Now feel your throat and neck. Feel your arms from shoulders to elbows, elbows to wrists, and wrist to fingers. Feel your hands. Now feel only your right hand. Now only your left hand. Right. Left. Feel both hands as sensation.

What are you aware of in this moment? Things like sensations will come and go, but as sensations change, they uncover an Awareness that never changes. Be the unchanging Awareness.

As Awareness, feel your chest and belly. Back. Pelvis. Legs. Feet.

Feel your entire body as very large. Now feel yourself as very small. Large. Small. This doesn't need to make sense, but in this moment become both small and large. Be both small and large.

Sensations will come and go, but each sensation points to your unchanging Awareness.

As Awareness, remember something that makes you happy. What is someone or something you love, something you love to do, or something that makes you laugh? Perhaps remember a time when you laughed so hard that you had tears streaming down your cheeks. Fill in the details of this person, object, or event that makes you happy by noticing your senses. What does this person, place, or thing look like, sound like, and smell like? What are the tastes associated with this happy scene? What are the sensations of your body in this scene?

Invite happiness into your body in this moment. Where do you feel happiness? Does it have a color? What are all the ways that happiness manifests in your being in this moment? Simply invite, acknowledge, and observe happiness.

Now, if it feels safe, I invite you to remember or imagine what it feels like to be disappointed. If that doesn't feel safe, you might choose a different emotion like boredom. Fill in the details of this scene in your head using your senses. What are the sights, smells, sounds, tastes, and sensations? Simply witness how this emotion feels in your body. Notice all the ways this emotion affects your being.

Now let go of disappointment or boredom and pick up happiness again. Remember the scene of happiness in your head. Now let go of happiness and remember disappointment or boredom. Happiness again. Disappointment or boredom. Now feel both simultaneously. Feel them together at the same time. Feel the part of you that is large enough to feel both emotions, the part of you that is larger than emotion.

In your mind, repeat the phrase "Though I have emotions, I am larger than emotions. Each emotion is pointing me to Awareness."

Bring your attention back to your body on the floor. Remember your Inner Sanctuary. Remember your Sankalpa if you had one. When you hear me count down from five (or ring the bell), that will signal the end of the Yoga Nidra practice. Through your practice of Awareness through emotions, you'll have the power to respond effectively to the emotions that visit you in your life.

5, 4, 3, 2, 1 (or ring the bell).

Yoga Nidra is over.

CHAPTER SEVEN

STEP 6: WITNESS THOUGHTS

How to Observe Your Mind

The French philosopher René Descartes proclaimed, "I think, therefore I am." Thanks, René, for creating the textbook definition of identifying with thoughts, that one's proof of existence lies within the ability to think. Descartes is not alone in this philosophy. At a fundamental level, most people believe that they are a thinking mind. Not so in Yoga Nidra, where thoughts are something to witness (and not be)—a philosophy that predates Descartes by thousands of years.

One's existence doesn't start and stop with the mind. Knowing your True Self isn't a philosophical or intellectual exercise. It's a felt experience. Yoga Nidra is the perfect practice to help you experience your True Self by training you to witness your thoughts, the product of the thinking mind. To witness thoughts, you must first be able to see your thoughts as separate from your observer self, your Awareness. That might sound like thinking about thinking. But with a little practice, you'll soon begin to feel yourself as the observer who happens to be witnessing thoughts the same way you can witness emotions, body, and sensations. This perspective comes relatively quickly once you welcome your thoughts and observe them rather than trying to control them.

Many people who try to practice meditation complain that it's too difficult, that their mind is simply too active. But in Yoga Nidra, the goal isn't to control thoughts but to simply watch them. They're just another interesting facet of your humanity that give you an avenue to practice Awareness.

You've probably heard the saying "What you resist, persists." Well, that's certainly true with thoughts. As often as you attempt to control your thoughts, they seem to want to pester you even more. For example, the more you try to resist thinking about the Brooklyn Blackout Cake at your favorite bakery, the more those tempting thoughts find themselves in your head. To witness thoughts, you must simply allow them free passage to come and go. I explain this process to my new meditation students through an analogy I call the Thought Factory.

You've just been hired as a supervisor to oversee thoughts at the Thought Factory. Your only job is to watch the conveyor belt. You're not trying to fix anything, not trying to change anything, and certainly not supposed to touch anything. Your boss puts you in front of a conveyer belt, and you must simply watch as it moves. Your gaze is fixed forward. Pretty soon, a thought comes along the conveyor belt. Though it might look tantalizing, your job is just to allow it to come and go. If you pick it up, you'll hold up production. Here's the thing: If you stop picking up the thoughts, the production gets done quicker, until there are fewer and fewer thoughts being sent your way. And when they do come, you're skilled at just watching them come and go.

What This Practice Does for You

The practice of witnessing your thoughts untangles your identity from your thinking mind. Your mind is part of the Vijnanamaya kosha (which also includes beliefs, prejudices, archetypes, and even the unconscious) and is a part of your being that you can practice being aware of.

Scientists estimate that more than 95 percent of our behavior could be based on beliefs and programming coming from the unconscious mind. Yoga Nidra offers a tremendous opportunity to access your unconscious mind, where you can insert powerful, positive programming using deep Awareness through your Sankalpa. This is one of the ways that Yoga Nidra has helped artists, students, and athletes perform at an elite level, and it's one of the ways that Yoga Nidra can help you manifest all the things you'd like to see in your life.

The mind is perhaps the most difficult layer to learn to observe objectively because it's constantly interpreting all the information it receives, organizing it, and calling that reality. There's an inherent problem with the mind thinking that it's got a corner on the market to reality, because the mind itself is constantly changing. You know what I mean: *LeBron is the best basketball player who ever lived and that's truth! Wait, no, it's Jordan . . .*

The Vijnanamaya kosha is defined as "illusion of the mind." The name points to the fact that the mind is not our reality but an illusion of it. Ultimately, through observing your thoughts, you'll experience yourself not as thoughts but as Awareness experiencing itself as thoughts in the present moment. Awareness exists only in the present moment. Time is the product of the mind, which is always labeling things as having happened or as yet to happen. Abstract concepts such as time might help us get to work when we're supposed to be there, but it can unfortunately also rob us from being present. If Awareness had a hand clock, it might simply have the word "now" in place of the numbers.

Speaking of timelessness, it's very common during Yoga Nidra to feel as though time has stopped. A 30-minute Yoga Nidra practice might feel like 10 minutes or an hour. This is because when you practice Awareness, you're only in the present and time doesn't have the same effect on your mind. The same could be said of intense or dramatic events. Time seems to stop the moment you meet the love of your life, see a loved one be born or pass away, or have a brush with death. Yoga Nidra is a way of experiencing this same kind of fierce presence—except without a trip to the emergency room. Being so focused on the present and learning to see your mind for what it is doesn't make you mindless; it makes you mindful.

5-MINUTE MEDITATION SCRIPT

To begin this Yoga Nidra practice, start by breathing in through your nose and sighing out through your mouth a few times. If you have a Sankalpa, repeat it now as a specific, positive, and present statement of truth. Fill in the details of your Inner Sanctuary using your senses.

Simply notice any thoughts you're experiencing at this moment. Simply witness them.

Feel your face, mouth, eyes, ears, and nose. Feel your entire head. Feel your neck, chest. Feel your arms. Feel only your left arm, only right. Left. Right. Feel both arms. Sensations change, revealing constant Awareness. Be Awareness. Feel your pelvis, legs, feet. Feel your entire body. Sensations change, revealing constant Awareness. Be Awareness.

Allow your body to rest comfortably on the floor. Visualize yourself walking down a hallway. Step by step, you're moving down the hallway. There's a door off to your left. Go inside a room where you are alone and comfortable. It's your own personal movie theater. As you sit, the lights dim. Projected onto a screen are all your thoughts. Without critique, merely watch them. Are they fast or slow? What is the subject? Do they evoke emotions, memories, or words? Remember, if anything arises that you prefer not to work with, you're always welcome to go back to your Inner Sanctuary. Otherwise, merely witness your thoughts.

Repeat in your mind, "Though I have thoughts, I am much bigger than my thoughts. Witnessing my thoughts reveals my Awareness."

Now feel your body lying on the floor. Revisit your Inner Sanctuary. Repeat your Sankalpa or repeat, "Though I have thoughts, I am much bigger than my thoughts. Witnessing my thoughts reveals my Awareness."

When you hear me count down from five (or ring the bell), that will signal the end of the Yoga Nidra practice.

5, 4, 3, 2, 1 (or ring the bell).

Yoga Nidra is over.

Get Started

Record either the short or long meditation (or both) in this chapter. Choose a time and place where you are least likely to be disturbed. Prepare your Yoga Nidra nest as usual, making sure you have everything handy that you might need for your practice. Before playing back the script, set aside about 5 minutes for the "There Is" meditation. I learned this meditation, which helps us practice being an objective observer to what's going on internally and externally, from yoga teacher Donna Farhi.

Sit or lie down, close your eyes, and simply begin to witness whatever arises in your Awareness with the phrase "There is." For example, in your mind, you might say, "There is the sensation of the body on the floor. There is the sound of the dog scratching at the door. There is anxiousness. There is a thought about work," and continue this way for five minutes. The idea is to preface whatever you are aware of in the moment with the phrase "There is."

There are two caveats to this practice: First, nothing is good or bad. It's all just information. In that vein, avoid making any sort of assessment about what pops into your Awareness and try to be as objective as possible. Instead of thinking, "There is some god-awful racket coming from across the street!" you might try something more neutral like, "There is sound across the street."

Second, avoid using pronouns like *I*, *me*, or *my*. Instead of thinking, "*I* hear the dog, *I* feel pressure on my back, or *I* am thinking about work," you would note, "There is the sound of the dog, there is the sensation of the back on the floor, there is a thought about work." This might seem a little forced and banal, but it actually serves a pretty sophisticated purpose: It helps change your entire object/subject paradigm. Instead of being something that is subject to what is happening internally or externally, you realize that it's all just objective information. This helps dissolve the false barrier between your body and your thoughts, bringing you into the larger realm of Awareness itself.

If your mind tends to race or wander in a meditation, this particular meditation is a good practice for you. You might want to try it regularly. Remember, in Yoga Nidra, you don't need to try to change or control your thinking. In this meditation, you are merely observing your thoughts with the phrase "There is." It might go like this: "There is a thought of this. Now there is a thought of that. Now there is another thought of this." Soon you'll find yourself witnessing the thinking without judging yourself for having an active mind (like most human beings). If your mind wanders, come back to the practice with, "There is wandering mind."

Once you've completed the "There Is" meditation, move on with your Yoga Nidra practice.

Reflect on Your Practice

As your Yoga Nidra practice concludes, take a moment to breathe deeply a few times into your body, slowly move your fingers and toes, and gently roll over to one side and rest in that position for a few moments. As you come up to a seated position, you may choose to repeat your Sankalpa a few times to yourself if you used one. You may also wish to repeat, "Though I have thoughts, I am much bigger than my thoughts. Witnessing my thoughts reveals my Awareness."

When you're ready, write down your immediate responses to the practice in your journal. As always, I encourage you to write freely and simply get the words out without attempting to make them sound eloquent. You can also respond to some or all of these questions in your journal:

- If you had one, what was your Sankalpa?

- How did time feel during your practice? Did your practice seem to pass quickly or slowly?

- Did you stay awake, or did you fall asleep? Did you find yourself drifting between waking and dreaming?

- Did you find it easy or difficult to witness your thoughts?

- What was your experience of witnessing your thoughts? Did your body react to your thoughts? What were all the ways your thoughts affected your being?

- Did you see images, see flashes of semi-formed thoughts, or experience memories?

- Did emotions arise?

- What were you most aware of during your practice?

✐ Did you hear words in your head or gain any unforeseen insight?

Images are like little mental packages that exist in the deeper regions of the mind and may speak to some of the unconscious things that play out in our waking life. Once, after I led a friend through a Yoga Nidra practice, I asked her if she experienced anything. "Not really," she said. "I just saw a quick picture of my dad resting on a bunch of rubble."

That's a perfect example of how an image may find its way into your practice. While you don't need to tease meaning from the images that present themselves, if you were to then begin inquiring about how those images sparked feelings, emotions, thoughts, memories, or sensations, you may gain some insight. Still, your job isn't to try to decode the images, because the work happens through Awareness. Having said that, images might be giving you a message that could be helpful in waking life, so just notice them.

As always, if you found that it was difficult to connect to your thoughts or felt that your thoughts themselves were actually so active that they got in the way of actually being able to witness them, don't worry; it's completely normal. One of the important reasons you record these scripts for yourself is so that you can listen to them several times. Your experience for each practice will be different because your mind will be in a different place and your level of Awareness will deepen with each session.

If you find that you fell asleep during this practice, you're not alone. The work you are performing in Yoga Nidra often works on a level that is too profound for the conscious mind to handle, especially in these deeper layers like the mind. It's as if our Awareness is shutting down the mind's operations for a while to do some internal maintenance deep in the system somewhere. Awareness, which is always paying attention regardless of whether we are asleep or not, anesthetizes the conscious mind for the work and reboots it when it's all done.

Full Meditation Script

Welcome to Yoga Nidra. Lie down and make yourself as comfortable as possible. Give yourself a slow breath in through the nose and out through the mouth with a sigh. Let go of any tension you might have.

If you wish to have a Sankalpa, repeat it now as a specific, positive, and present statement of truth. If you wish to use your Inner Sanctuary in this practice, give yourself a moment to fill in the details of your sanctuary using your senses.

Start by bringing your attention to everything that feels external to you in this moment: sounds, smells, temperature, and so on. Now bring your attention to whatever feels internal: emotions, thoughts, and internal sensations. Welcome whatever you experience, either internally or externally, simply as information. Recognize it for what it is and merely be the observer of it. Now, be aware of everything external and internal simultaneously. In this moment, be Awareness itself, experiencing itself as whatever you're aware of in this moment.

Bring your attention to the sensation of your face: your mouth, eyes, ears, and nose. Feel your scalp: the top of your head and back of your head. Feel your face and scalp simultaneously. Feel your entire head. Feel the sensation of your neck and throat. Your collarbones and chest. Feel your arms: shoulders, elbows, forearms, wrists, and hands. Feel only your left arm, now only your right arm. Left. Right. Feel both arms.

While sensation changes, it reveals that which is never changing: Awareness. Be Awareness itself. As Awareness, experience yourself as belly, back. Now feel your pelvis. Feel your legs. Feel your feet. Feel your entire body as sensation. Feel your entire body. Sensations may change, but Awareness never does. Be Awareness.

I invite you to go with me on a mental journey. Allow your body to rest comfortably on the floor and visualize yourself walking down a hallway. Step by step, you're moving down a long hallway. You feel your arms moving at your side; you feel your legs moving as you move deeper and deeper down a hallway. Eventually, you find a door off to your left. Go inside the door into a room where you are alone and comfortable.

The room is set up like your own personal movie theater. There's a beautiful, cozy chair in the middle of the room, and as you sit down, the lights dim and you see projected onto a screen all the thoughts you are having in this moment. Your job is not to critique or control these thoughts but merely watch them. Watch your thoughts as they play out on the screen. Are they moving fast or slow? Are they in color or black-and-white? What is the subject of the thoughts? Do the thoughts evoke any emotions? Do the thoughts evoke memories or words? Do they evoke other thoughts? Nothing is supposed to happen or not supposed to happen, and remember, if anything arises that you prefer not to work with, you're always welcome to go back to your Inner Sanctuary. Otherwise, merely witness your thinking and notice all the ways your thoughts are affecting your being. You are not responsible for changing or controlling your thoughts; you're witnessing your thoughts. There is no value to thoughts.

Now visualize yourself getting up out of the seat and walking to the door and going back out into the hallway. Notice that your thoughts are still playing. Walk back up the hallway, the direction from which you came. Repeat in your mind, "Though I have thoughts, I am much bigger than my thoughts. Witnessing my thoughts reveals my Awareness."

As Awareness, experience yourself walking back up the hallway and finally rejoining your body lying on the floor. Feel your body lying on the floor.

Revisit your Inner Sanctuary if you wish. Repeat your Sankalpa or the phrase "Though I have thoughts, I am much bigger than my thoughts. Witnessing my thoughts reveals my Awareness."

When you hear me count down from five (or ring the bell), that will signal the end of the Yoga Nidra practice.

5, 4, 3, 2, 1 (or ring the bell).
Yoga Nidra is over.

STEP 7:
TAP INTO JOY

How to Tap into Your Joy

Tapping into your joy means practicing daily happiness and
pleasure. It's about learning to see the myriad things around you
all the time that can cause you joy. However, your joy is not actually dependent on events and circumstances, and it's accessible
whenever you wish. In Yoga Nidra, joy is found beyond the mind.
When you have the know-how, there is little or no effort to connect to this part of your being. Eventually, with practice, you won't
need a trigger to feel this joy. You'll simply *be* joy. This limitless joy
is your True Nature.

Despite whatever pain you may have experienced or whatever
scars are on your heart, you have unfettered joy waiting to be
dusted off. This joy is your essence. It has always existed the same
way you have always existed. Learning to tap into the joy that

is always with you opens your heart to inexhaustible prana, or energy. For example, in his audio program *Clear Mind, Wild Heart,* writer and poet David Whyte shares a story about a time when he felt utterly exhausted by his work for a nonprofit. He asked his friend Brother David Steindl-Rast (a Catholic Benedictine monk) half-jokingly, "What's the antidote to exhaustion?" His friend looked at him for a moment and then responded with something Whyte found life-changing: "The antidote to exhaustion isn't necessarily rest. It's wholeheartedness."

Whyte realized that, at that moment in his life, his heart was yearning for him to devote himself to poetry instead of the work he was doing for the nonprofit. From that moment forward, he started letting go of what didn't tap into his joy so that he could put all of his energies into what did. Whyte has since become a world-renowned poet, speaker, and author. That's not to say you need to give up the work you do, of course; you can begin tapping into joy by simply noticing when you smile or laugh, remembering what you love, doing the things you enjoy wholeheartedly, and of course practicing Yoga Nidra.

Learning to tap into your limitless joy can be fun and easy. It's the momentary joys in life that reveal your unchanging joy, the feeling of your True Self. Make it a regular practice to notice the things you love about life. You have an immense power to create or interpret your reality, and focusing on what brings you joy and what you want to see in your life is key to feeling in love with life. If you adopt a Hobbesian approach to life, that it is "nasty, brutish, and short," you'll find endless proof to support that view. But if you adopt an *It's a Wonderful Life* approach, you'll find just as much proof.

If you get to create your reality, why not make it as beautiful as possible by noticing all of its joy, love, and sensuality? As you allow joy, love, and sensuality to become regular features in your life, you'll soon find that your entire life becomes an expression of this joy. Doing this regularly will also prime you to invite these elements into your Yoga Nidra practice.

What This Practice Does for You

Your complete happiness and sensuality lie within the subtle layer of your being called the Anandamaya kosha (the bliss body). This kind of joy isn't momentary happiness that comes and goes; rather, it is the unlimited bliss you experience as your True Self. However, learning to witness life's momentary joys helps prepare you to feel your True Self's natural state of limitless joy. As I mentioned in chapter 3, the mind makes little distinction between what plays out on a screen, in your mind, or in real life. Your brain doesn't differentiate between what's real and imagined, so visualizing what makes you happy can have the same effect as actually experiencing it.

While our True Nature is joy, ironically, we have been programmed to be pretty negative. In fact, humanity's survival may very well have depended on it. Think about it: You're less likely to jump into a shallow lake if you think you might hit jagged rocks at the bottom. Therefore, finding your joy through Yoga Nidra and similar practices is a process that essentially rewires the brain from its negative default to inhabiting our birthright to be unfailingly happy. It's the kind of happiness you don't have to wait around for. No one's going to give it to you, and it's not tied to any event. Like it or not, no one and nothing is responsible for your happiness. You must decide to see what is joyful around you and make it a regular practice to invite joy into your life.

Several years ago, my friend Kim's dad, Warren, suffered a serious spinal cord injury. He's confined to a wheelchair, has very limited movement in his arms and legs, and requires daily help from nurses, especially after his wife and caretaker passed away. A while back, Kim and I were staying at Warren's house along with Kim's sister and two daughters. Warren and I were sharing a room, and as we were tucking into our beds, he began to muse about how many of his friends enjoy luxuries like big houses, boats, and cars. With tears in his eyes, he said, "You know, when I see my daughters and my granddaughters, I can't help but feel like I've won in life. I've won!" Warren sat there in the dark with a wide grin on his face. He didn't say a thing about any of the challenges that beset his life and chose only to see the joy.

5-MINUTE MEDITATION SCRIPT

To begin this Yoga Nidra practice, start with a cleansing sigh. Repeat your Sankalpa to yourself.

Become aware of your body as sensation. Remember what it feels like to float in a warm bath. It's warm, comfortable, and relaxing. Feel your head, neck, arms, chest, belly, back, legs, and feet. Everything is comfortable, floating in the warm water.

Visualize a scene of yourself feeling happy. Experience the shapes and colors or textures, smells, sounds, and tastes. What does your body feel in this moment?

How does happiness feel? Allow the feelings to rise to the surface. Where do you feel those emotions in your body? Welcome the feelings and emotions. Do these feelings evoke colors, images, or memories? Simply witness the emotion and feeling. Rest in the feeling and emotion. Release the vision and stay with the feeling. What is observing the feeling and emotion? Be the observer.

Go with me on a mental journey. Walk up a mountain path, higher and higher. At the top of the mountain, there is a table. On it is something that represents joy, love, or pleasure. Pick it up. Put the object down. There is another object that represents pain, sadness, or discomfort. Don't choose something too difficult. Pick up this object. Now hold both objects simultaneously. What is the part of you that can hold pleasure and pain simultaneously? Joy isn't dependent upon events and circumstances. Place both objects on the table. Walk down the mountain the way you came.

> Feel your body lying on the floor. Because you've prac-
> ticed Awareness through feeling happy, you'll be able to live
> life more joyfully.
>
> When you hear me count down from five (or ring the
> bell), that will signal the end of the Yoga Nidra practice.
>
> 5, 4, 3, 2, 1 (or ring the bell).
>
> Yoga Nidra is over.

Get Started

Record either the short or long meditation (or both) in this chap-
ter. Prepare for your Yoga Nidra practice by choosing a time and
a place to practice when you are the least likely to be disturbed.
Arrange all of your props, including your Yoga Nidra journal.
Remember to put your phone in airplane mode and place your
"Do Not Disturb" sign on the door if you use one.

Before you practice, do something that makes you feel sensual,
like give yourself a little massage, rub some nice-smelling oil on
your skin, or eat a piece of chocolate. Practice focusing on the joy
it gives you as you do it. Then, in your Yoga Nidra journal, do the
following writing practice:

Set a timer for 11 minutes and then start jotting down everything that brings you joy, big and small, without stopping or
editing what you write. You could write this as a "love letter to
life" or simply make a list of all the things you find joyful.

If you choose the letter, write it as if you were writing it to a lover.
It might read something like, "Dear life, the way you sweep me off
my feet every time I look up and see yet another mind-blowing
sunset, reminding me of your infinite beauty, brings me such joy.
Thank you so much for all those joyful notes you send me in the
form of little delights, like walking by that café yesterday and hearing
my favorite jazz song wafting out into the streets, like the jasmine
bush you charmed me with on my walk yesterday after work, and like
night's soothing bath with a good book after work . . ."

If you're not wild about writing a love letter, simply list all the things that bring you joy and make sure you start each sentence with the phrase "I find joy in . . ." It might go like this: "I find joy in coffee and toast in the morning. I find joy in spending time with my dog. I find joy in a fast and easy commute to work. I find joy in the taste of chocolate cake. I find joy in getting massages. I find joy hiking in the mountains . . ." If you get stuck and don't know what to write, just keep writing the phrase "I find joy" until something pops up and the list begins again.

Then, when you're ready, settle in for your Yoga Nidra practice and play back your recording.

Reflect on Your Practice

As your Yoga Nidra practice concludes, take a moment to breathe deeply a few times into your body, slowly move your fingers and toes, and gently roll over to one side. Rest in that position for a few moments and then sit up. As you come to a seated position, take a moment and notice how you feel after focusing on joy.

In your Yoga Nidra journal, write down your immediate responses to the practice. As always, don't worry about making it sound good. Just do your best to get your ideas on paper. You can also respond to some or all of these questions in your journal:

⌀ What was your experience of feeling joy like in this Yoga Nidra practice?

⌀ Did you stay awake, or did you fall asleep? Did you find yourself drifting between waking and dreaming?

⌀ What did you discover about the source of your joy?

⌀ Did you find it easy or difficult to invite joyfulness into your practice and why?

⌀ How do you feel about the idea of being responsible for your own happiness?

Once, during a Sanskrit lecture, the speaker described the notion in yoga philosophy that all the love and joy we have inside of us exists before we ever feel it. He said that we misappropriate our love and joy when we feel that another person "makes" us feel loved or happy. I immediately thought, "That's the most unromantic, wet blanket I've ever heard." For a moment, my heart fell, thinking that all that brings me love and joy was my own invention and not some beautiful outside and mysterious force lighting me up with these emotions.

Then it dawned on me that the power of all the love and joy I possessed wasn't dependent upon another person or thing. Suddenly, I felt like I was handed a blank check for love and joy that would allow me to feel these emotions anytime I wanted to, 24/7, regardless of circumstances. I recognized that all the people I love are the beneficiaries of something that already and always exists. It can exist whether or not they know it or even reciprocate it. It's like when I tell my toddler, "I love you," and he responds with, "Well, I don't love you." I say, "That's OK. I still love you." I know from his sweet kisses on my cheeks that he truly does love me, but the concept is the same: I don't have to wait for anyone to love me for me to feel love or joy. The fact is, I just love and feel joy. I can draw on my limitless resource of love and joy anytime I want it by simply thinking about my son's sweet face wide with laughter, and instantly I'm filled with love and joy. It's happening now.

We can tap our eternal source of joy and love simply by remembering those things we love. The joy we feel temporarily reminds us of and reveals our blissful essence.

Full Meditation Script

Welcome to Yoga Nidra. Lie down and make yourself as comfortable as possible. Give yourself a few deep breaths, breathing in through your nose and sending your breath out through your mouth with a sigh. Release any tension you may have.

If you wish to use a Sankalpa, repeat it now in your mind as a specific, positive, and present statement of truth. As always, simply invite, acknowledge, and observe anything that arises in your Awareness.

Feel your body on the floor. Become aware of your body as sensation. Remember what it feels like to float in a warm bath. Start by feeling your head floating in the bath or resting on the edge of the tub. It's warm, comfortable, and relaxing. Feel your neck meet the warm water. Feel your arms completely relaxed and floating in the warm water. Feel both of your arms simultaneously. Feel your chest and belly move as you breathe, making slight movements in the warm water. Feel your back resting in the warm water. Feel your legs and feet floating in the water. Everything is comfortable, floating in the water. Feel your entire body—relaxed, alive, and sensual. Feel your entire body. Though sensations change, Awareness remains the same. Be the unchanging Awareness experiencing itself as the body.

Remember or imagine a time when you felt happy. Fill in the details of this scene using all of your senses. Notice shapes, colors, or textures. Notice smells. Sounds. Tastes. Are there other people, animals, or special objects around you? What does your body feel in this moment?

What does it feel like to feel when it's happy? Allow those feelings and emotions to rise to the surface in this moment. Where do you feel those emotions in your body? Welcome the feelings and emotions. It's natural to feel this. Do these feelings evoke colors, images, or memories? Now simply witness the emotion and feeling. Rest in the feeling and emotion.

Now let go of the memory or the visualization of the scene and merely stay with the feeling and emotion. Simply notice how it feels. Notice that the feeling was right there, close to the surface. All you had to do was remember what it felt like, and immediately it was there. This feeling is within you always. What is observing the feeling and emotion? Be the observer of this joy. Notice if or how this feeling lingers or expands.

Allow your body to rest on the floor and go with me on a mental journey. You're walking up a mountain path, each step bringing you higher and higher. Your body feels alive, strong, and energized as you continue to climb up the mountain. The air is fresh and clean and fills your lungs. At the top of the mountain, there is a table, and on it is something that brings or represents joy, love, or pleasure. Pick up this object and hold it in your hands. What does it feel like? Put the object down.

There is another object that brings or represents pain, sadness, or discomfort. You don't need to choose something that is very difficult. Pick up this object and feel it in your hands. Now put down that object and pick up the object that brings you joy, love, or pleasure. Put that object down and pick up the other. Now pick up both objects and feel them both in your hands simultaneously. What is the part of you that can hold pleasure and pain simultaneously? Feel the joy of being. Feel the joy that isn't dependent upon events and circumstances. Place both objects on the table. Walk down the mountain the way you came.

Feel your body again lying on the floor. Because you've been able to practice Awareness through feeling joy, you'll be able to live life more fully from this place. You'll see joy in everything you do.

When you hear me count down from five (or ring the bell), that will signal the end of the Yoga Nidra practice.

5, 4, 3, 2, 1 (or ring the bell).

Yoga Nidra is over.

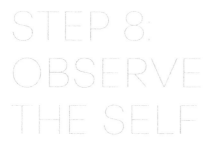

CHAPTER NINE

STEP 8: OBSERVE THE SELF

How to See Your True Self

As we move on to step 8, let's bypass some confusion with a brief explanation: When the word *Self* is capitalized, it is referring to our True Self. When it is lowercased, it is referring to the ego or the parts of us that we might tend to identify with but which are ultimately inadequate to express our full identity. As you've learned, Yoga Nidra talks about the *self* in the form of the koshas, or layers: body, energy, emotions, thoughts, and bliss. The Self, on the other hand, is everything about us that is eternal and doesn't change; it is synonymous with *Awareness*. Your Self existed before you were born and will exist when your body dies. Self is the Source that the Gayatri Mantra, which I shared on page 14, talks about. It may sound a bit like a riddle, but Yoga Nidra is a method to leverage the self as a tool to illuminate the Self.

To become familiar with the Self, you must learn how to arrive at being the observer of all the elements of your ego rather than identifying with and reacting to them. One of my favorite ways to do this is to meditate and be like the supervisor at the Thought Factory from chapter 7. As you meditate, your only job is to watch the elements of your ego (in this case, thoughts) simply come and go. If ever a particularly tantalizing thought comes down the conveyor belt and you pick it up, try it on like a new coat, and run around town all day pointing to it, you got caught up in the self and lost your observer, your Self.

I can tell you from experience that the upper management at the Thought Factory is very understanding and won't fire you over such behavior. Otherwise they'd have to hire a new supervisor every 10 seconds. Eventually you start to become good at watching your thoughts, body, energy, emotions, and everything else until you become adept at processing these things. It becomes easier, then, for what seem like distractions to come and go.

There's a curious thing that happens next. I notice it often during Yoga Nidra, other meditations, and sometimes while I'm living daily life. It's a feeling like a veil has dropped away or a switch has been flipped, and my identity shifts. All of a sudden, I'm the observer watching my thoughts rather than thinking my thoughts. I'm watching my body feel sensation rather than equating my being as a body that feels sensation. The thoughts and sensations keep going along their merry way, but I feel perched above it all. This is the observation of Self.

What This Practice Does for You

Concentration, relaxation, and playing with opposites (being simultaneously aware of two opposing things) are a few essential tools used in Yoga Nidra to help you learn to observe the Self. The Yoga Nidra process begins by moving scattered attention into a well-honed focus that's welcoming, recognizing, and witnessing all things that are presented to you. You might be asked to begin concentrating on the sounds in the room and then narrow your focus to your Sankalpa and Inner Sanctuary. The scope zeroes in even more as you sense your body and yet again as you do a body scan and other aspects of the practice.

Once you've achieved this very pointed attention, anything that spontaneously enters your field—like an idea for tonight's dinner, for example—will feel like an intruder. You'll recognize it as something different from what you were previously experiencing as you invite, acknowledge, and observe it. The part that can now see that thought as an intruder is the observer, the Self.

Previously, this same thought would have been another thing that was spreading your attention around. Now, in a state of concentration, you can objectively see this thought as something that's interrupting focus, this Awareness. This process of refining your focus to a singular concentration helps you experience yourself as the observer and notice your Self. Many, perhaps even most, of the popular meditation styles employ concentration as the pathway to the observer.

As I've mentioned previously, Yoga Nidra differs from most meditation styles with its emphasis on relaxation. Relaxed Awareness is one of Yoga Nidra's superpowers. The world created by the mind softens a little as you unwind, especially if you arrive at the state of consciousness between waking and dreaming. Like the ugly duckling finally coming to see itself as the swan, sometimes you have to rest your mind a little to abandon previously held identities and see your True Self.

Like the Gayatri Mantra suggests, everything that exists is part of you, and you're a part of everything. This is Self. The mind (the ego-self) tends to fracture our wholeness into opposite parts—this or that, right or wrong. But when you ask your consciousness to see these parts as integral and not separate, you're actually using the self to experience the Self. Truly, it's not a riddle but an experience you will come to know with practice.

5-MINUTE MEDITATION SCRIPT

To begin this Yoga Nidra practice, breathe in through your nose and out through your mouth with a sigh, and release any tension. Repeat your Sankalpa and visualize your Inner Sanctuary.

Feel your face. Scalp. Top and back of your head. Now the entire head. Feel your neck, collarbones, chest, arms, belly, back, pelvis, legs, and feet. Feel your entire body as sensation. Sensation may change, but Awareness never does. Be Awareness.

As Awareness, imagine yourself inside your body looking out. Now imagine yourself outside your body looking in. Inside looking out. Outside looking in. In this moment, you're both inside looking out and outside looking in.

Take a journey with me. Leave your body lying on the floor and expand larger than the room, building, city, continent, world, and Universe. You're as large as the Universe. In this space, you feel very comfortable. There is no up or down, right or left. There is no right or wrong. There is no past or future. It's the perfect moment of now. You can see everything in the Universe as yourself. You can be as small as the smallest particle and as large as the largest galaxy.

Zoom in and look at your body lying on the floor. See your entire life from beginning to end. You see your life as a beautiful and interesting expression of your Universal Self. As the Universe, you can direct and organize things how you wish. Notice how the life of the person who is lying on the floor is playing out. Simply notice the life of the person lying on the floor.

Now feel yourself shift from the large Universal Self to become as small as a galaxy, world, continent, city, building, and room. Come to rest in the body lying on the floor.

Feel your body. Revisit your Inner Sanctuary if you wish. Repeat your Sankalpa. When you hear me count down from five (or ring the bell), that will signal the end of the Yoga Nidra practice.

5, 4, 3, 2, 1 (or ring the bell).

Yoga Nidra is over.

Get Started

Record either the short or long meditation (or both) in this chapter. So far you've practiced using your senses to experience Awareness. To listen to your Self, it's time to go beyond your senses and be at one with all things. The *Yoga Sutras* are an ancient text that is the source of much yoga philosophy. In part, it outlines the eight-limbed path of yoga, which is the path of knowing the Self. The eight-limbed path covers the following:

How you treat the world (Yama)

Noticing your inner world, cleanliness, and contentedness (Niyama)

Awareness of body with yoga postures (Asana)

Awareness of energy with breath control (Pranayama)

Disassociate from your senses (Pratyahara)

Focused concentration (Dharana)

Deep meditation (Dhyana)

Being at one with all things (Samadhi)

The last one—Samadhi—is to constantly be aware of Self. Though it may seem lofty, we all experience this type of awareness throughout our lives from time to time, usually when we are fiercely present in one of the intense encounters life may offer. Yoga Nidra, however, is a way of practicing this fierce presence in conditions we set up for ourselves rather than waiting for life to do it for us.

Two practices from the eight-limbed path that can prepare you to observe the Self in Yoga Nidra are Bhramari Breath (to withdraw from the senses) and mantra meditation (for deep concentration). Bhramari Breath (sometimes called Bumblebee Breath) can be done several ways, but you'll do it lying down as you prepare for your Yoga Nidra practice.

Set yourself up the way you typically do for Yoga Nidra, including making arrangements not to be disturbed and grabbing your journal. For this breathing exercise, I suggest using either an eye mask, scarf, or bandanna to cover your eyes as well as earplugs to plug your ears.

Once your Yoga Nidra nest is set up, ear plugs in, and eye mask on, lie down as you would to practice Yoga Nidra, cushions under knees and all. Once you're lying down, give yourself a few deep Ujjayi Breaths (see page 46). Next, take a big inhale, and instead of exhaling, hum a long, slow hum until you run out of breath. Breathe in and do it again. Continue for 7 to 10 rounds. Because your eyes are covered and ears are plugged, your senses will quickly draw inward. All your attention will be on the sound of your own voice in your head. You may choose whichever humming tone you'd like. You may even switch tones. Once you finish doing 7 to 10 rounds, you'll feel very drawn in and ready to do the mantra meditation.

Mantra means to transcend your mind through a word or phrase. There are various yoga mantras such as *om mani padme hum*, but for this practice, I suggest you create a Sankalpa that is specific, positive, and present to use as your mantra. Repeat it in your mind several times for three or five minutes, and then start your Yoga Nidra practice.

Reflect on Your Practice

As your Yoga Nidra practice concludes, pause for a moment and open your Awareness to how your body feels. Give yourself a few deep breaths and take your time as you open your eyes and roll over onto one side. Rest in that position for a moment, and when you're ready, come back up to a seated position. If you used a Sankalpa for this practice, you may wish to repeat it now.

In your journal, write down your immediate responses to the practice, writing freely and without edits. As usual, just do a word dump onto the page. You can also respond to some or all of these questions in your journal:

- Did you notice the observer, the Self? What was that experience like?

- How would you describe the feeling of observing your self with the Self?

- How can becoming aware of the Self help you operate in your everyday life?

- What challenges did you face as you practiced noticing the Self, if any?

- Can you or did you gain insights from noticing your Self? If so, what are they?

If you found this practice difficult or confusing, don't worry. This is a process and a practice. This is about learning to find some sense of objectivity with the world your mind has created. Ultimately, it's not about abandoning or disparaging the ego-self on the way to knowing the True Self. Rather it's embracing the marriage of the two, our Both/And nature. Through one, you'll find the other and then live your life in a way that is practical and real.

You'll also just happen to see everything with wondrous Awareness and joy.

There's a great yoga myth that illustrates this perfectly and goes a little like this: In the beginning, there was Shiva, who represents pure consciousness, and Shakti, who is everything that is form and movement. Shiva has a third eye in the middle of his forehead that represents consciousness and watches Shakti. Shakti is always moving and dancing for Shiva. Together, they are the perfect balance and complete each other. Shakti is always interested in changing things up, so one day she dances around behind Shiva and covers his ever-watching third eye. For a split second, Universal consciousness ceases and there's only movement, causing an enormous explosion in the Universe. Shakti finds herself reeling through space separated from her lover, Shiva.

Shakti wanders, searching for Shiva and sensing him everywhere but can't see him. She feels lost and separate. Then one day she sits and meditates the way she's seen Shiva do. She begins to hear his voice speak to her. As she pays closer and closer attention, she hears him say, "Shakti. I am here. I've always been here. Nothing exists without me, the way nothing exists without you." At that, Shakti opens her eyes and no longer sees the trees, birds, and water—only Shiva in the form of all those things.

This is a beautiful story that maps our own experience of once being at one with the Universe, then being born and feeling separate from our Self, and then through the experience of our life coming back into the knowledge of our own wholeness, our Self.

Full Meditation Script

Welcome to Yoga Nidra. Lie down and make yourself as comfortable as possible. Give yourself a slow breath in through the nose and out through the mouth with a sigh. Let go of any tension.

If you wish to have a Sankalpa, repeat it now as a specific, positive, and present statement of truth. If you wish to use your Inner Sanctuary in this practice, give yourself a moment and fill in the details of your sanctuary using your senses.

Start by bringing your attention to the space outside of you; sense everything from your body out. Now bring your attention to the space inside of you; sense everything from your skin inward. Welcome whatever you experience, either internally or externally, simply as information. Now feel the space inside and outside of you simultaneously. Imagine your skin like one of the rings in a tree trunk, rings that extend eternally outward and eternally inward.

Bring your attention to the sensation of your face: your mouth, eyes, ears, and nose. Feel your scalp: the top of your head and back of your head. Feel your face and scalp simultaneously. Feel your entire head. Feel the sensation of your neck and throat. Your collarbones and chest. Feel your arms: shoulders, elbows, forearms, wrists, and hands. Feel only your left arm. Feel only your right arm. Left. Right. Feel both arms. While sensations change, they reveal that which is never changing: Awareness. Be Awareness itself. As Awareness, experience yourself as belly, back. Now feel your pelvis. Feel your legs. Feel your feet. Feel your entire body as sensation. Feel your entire body. Sensations may change, but Awareness never does. Be Awareness.

As Awareness, imagine yourself inside your body looking out. You can see all of the things in the room. You notice the walls, ceiling, and furniture. Now imagine yourself outside your body looking in. You can see your body's shape. You can see yourself breathing and resting on the floor. Now you're inside your body looking out again. Now you're outside your body looking in. In this moment, you're both inside looking out and outside looking in.

Take a journey with me. Leave your body lying comfortably on the floor and expand to become larger than the room, larger than the house or building you're in, larger than your city, continent, and larger than the world. You're larger than the galaxy. You're as large as the Universe. In this space, you feel very comfortable. There is no up or down, right or left. There is no right or wrong. There is no past or future. It's always a perfect moment of now. Everything simply is. You can see everything in the Universe as yourself. You can be as small as the smallest particle and as large as the largest galaxy.

As the Universe itself, zoom in and look at your body lying on the floor. You can see your entire life from beginning to end. You see your life as an intricate tapestry of events and people and a beautiful and interesting expression of your Universal Self. As the Universe, you can direct and organize things how you wish. Notice how the life of the person who is lying on the floor is playing out. Without the need to fix, change, or do anything, simply notice the life of the person lying on the floor.

Now feel yourself shift from the large Universal Self to become as small as a galaxy, as the world, the continent, the city, the house or building, the room, and now come to rest in the body lying on the floor.

Feel your body lying on the floor.

Revisit your Inner Sanctuary if you wish. Repeat your Sankalpa. When you hear me count down from five (or ring the bell), that will signal the end of the Yoga Nidra practice.

5, 4, 3, 2, 1 (or ring the bell).

Yoga Nidra is over.

CHAPTER TEN

STEP 9: VISUALIZE

How to Use Visualizations

Visualizations are scenes you evoke in your mind by using your senses. Your Inner Sanctuary is a good example of a visualization. Visualizations work with your unconscious mind to adjust ideas of what's possible and help you live a more fulfilled life with deeper Awareness. The truth is, many of our actions are the product of our unconscious mind, and as you learned earlier, our unconscious mind could even be responsible for 95 percent of the actions we take. Therefore, visualization is a powerful way to understand, decode, and even rewire your unconscious mind.

For most of us, seeing is believing. Remember how your brain doesn't differentiate very well between what you're visualizing and what's happening in real life? If you can see yourself succeeding, you can remove the unconscious blocks that prevent you from meeting your potential. Trust me, you are much more capable than you realize. But while visualizations can give you this deep personal insight, that's really not their function in our Yoga Nidra practice.

The purpose of visualization in this step of the 10-step method is to practice seeing all parts of yourself to gain Awareness. If in your Awareness through visualization you see that you could respond to some stimuli a bit better in your life, then great. That's a wonderful by-product of Awareness. Revealing something about your unconscious or gaining a message from your wise inner teacher could, in fact, be that tool that helps you become more aware.

Not all teachers use visualizations in Yoga Nidra, and those who do have their own takes—some simply invite the conscious mind to notice how it responds to concepts and phrases. For example, if you were to ask 10 people what their immediate response to the word "businessman" is, there would be 10 different responses. This kind of visualization reveals what kind of associations you may have and perhaps shows how they affect your waking life. Other types of visualizations in Yoga Nidra include graduated exposure to emotional triggers, connecting to spirit guides, noticing and rewiring beliefs around money, or visualizing optimal performance. I personally find visualizations effective in creating powerful action in a person's life through the practice of Awareness.

What This Practice Does for You

Visualizations in a Yoga Nidra practice help create a conversation between your conscious and unconscious mind. Like your conscious, or thinking, mind, your unconscious mind rests in the Vijnanamaya kosha. A good question might be how the conscious mind can be aware of the unconscious—isn't that the point, that it's *un*conscious? In Yoga Nidra, we go beyond the thinking mind to gain an Awareness that is broad enough to hold both conscious and unconscious mind alike. Yoga Nidra is like a handy bridge between the conscious and unconscious mind so there can be understanding and commerce between the two.

So much of what you believe about what's possible or what you deserve in the world comes from your unconscious. As you relax and graduate into deepening layers of Awareness through Yoga Nidra, you can reveal some of the unconscious programming that's running your life. This can be very illuminating to help to decode some of your unconscious actions and decisions like, for example, why you can never take a day off work even if you're sick or why you keep losing at Scrabble with your best friend even though you can spell the pants off them. I can't tell you why you don't think you deserve a day off or why you take a nosedive at Scrabble, but with continued Yoga Nidra practice, including visualization, you can gain some insight and put some positive programming into your unconscious mind.

Aiming for a seven-letter word on the triple-word score square? Have an important presentation to give at work? Want to nail your next job interview? Wondering if you could ever find the love of your life? Using visualizations is an easy and effective way to access or program your unconscious mind to bring your best self forward into conscious action. A lot of famous people have used visualization to bring their best selves forward, including Muhammad Ali, Will Smith, Jim Carrey, Billie Jean King, Oprah Winfrey, and Carli Lloyd, to name just a few. In an interview recorded in the *Harvard Business Review*, Greg Louganis chalks up his ability for success and focus during competition to his practice of visualization.

Maybe Olympic diving isn't your focus in life and what you'd love more than a gold medal is to learn to sleep well. Visualization through Yoga Nidra is a very powerful and effective way to help you achieve incredible sleep. One day a student came into Yoga Nidra class with desperation in her bloodshot eyes. "I haven't slept well in over six months and I'm going crazy. Can Yoga Nidra help that?" she pleaded. "You're in the right place," I assured her.

During practice, we visualized getting very relaxed and achieving deep, peaceful, and nourishing sleep. After class she told me that she did not fall asleep during the practice but was the most relaxed she had been in months. She came back to class a few days later and reported that on the night of that Yoga Nidra class, she'd been able to achieve the first good night of sleep in six months. This student is not alone. Unfortunately, inadequate sleep is very common, and something as simple as a visualization through Yoga Nidra is a natural and effective way to help.

Once you understand the principles of why visualizations work and how to use them, you can guide yourself through your own visualizations independent of your Yoga Nidra practice.

5-MINUTE MEDITATION SCRIPT

To begin this Yoga Nidra practice, start with a tension-releasing sigh. Repeat your Sankalpa and visualize your Inner Sanctuary using all your senses.

Feel your face. Scalp. Top and back of head. Entire head. Feel neck, collarbones, chest, arms, belly, back, pelvis, legs, and feet. Feel your entire body as sensation. Be Awareness.

Now take an inner journey down a hallway. Feel all your senses as you walk this hallway. You're on a journey to see a very wise person with an important message for you.

Notice a door off to your left. As you open the door, you see your thoughts. Witness thoughts. Close the door and walk down the hallway.

There's a door at the end of the hallway. You open it to see a wise person waiting for you. Who is the wisest person? This wise person loves you. This person knows you perhaps even better than you know yourself.

With a smile, your wise person says, "The very important thing about you that I wanted to tell you is . . ." Hear the first thing that comes. Pause for a moment and listen for the words to come. You might experience words, feelings, thoughts, emotions, or images. If the message doesn't come immediately, it will come eventually.

With a smile and a hug, you head back out the door and back up the way you came. You can return whenever you like. You hold the gift of the wise person's words in your heart.

Feel yourself walking back up the hallway. Check in with your thoughts. Now continue up the hallway.

Now feel your body. Remember your Sankalpa, Inner Sanctuary, and the wise words.

When you hear me count down from five (or ring the bell), that will signal the end of the Yoga Nidra practice.

5, 4, 3,2, 1 (or ring the bell).

Yoga Nidra is over.

Get Started

Record either the short or long meditation (or both) in this chapter. Set yourself up for Yoga Nidra as usual by arranging your Yoga Nidra nest and having everything you need close by. Since visualization happens on a level deeper than the mind, it's important to relax the mind as much as possible before you begin to get the most benefit. In other words, choose a time for this Yoga Nidra practice when you are normally relaxed and not overly stimulated.

One of my regular Yoga Nidra students felt frustrated because she often fell asleep during Yoga Nidra practice and felt like she missed the entire visualization. I reminded her that we are working on an even deeper level than the conscious mind so that even if she falls asleep, the visualization still takes effect. Nonetheless, she really wanted to be awake, so she drank four shots of espresso before practice. Yes, she stayed awake during the visualization, but she reported afterward that the only thing she was aware of was her pounding heart and racing agitation. She relented and gave up on the goal of trying to stay awake, and ironically, she has a much easier time staying awake. It wasn't until after she could allow herself to relax, come what may, that she finally experienced a very personal and meaningful message during the visualization.

Remember, visualizations can be cool and provide you with deep personal insight, but the purpose of the visualizations in the 10-step method is to practice seeing all parts of yourself to gain Awareness.

If, after practicing with the scripts in this chapter, you'd like to make your own visualizations for specific things you might need in your life, such as success with an event or project or seeking guidance from your inner teachers (like spirit guides, animal messengers, or a wiser version of yourself in the future), create your visualization the way you did your Sankalpa by making it specific, positive, and present. These three elements help you conceptualize your visualization using the language of your deep unconscious mind and that of your True Self.

When guiding yourself, take the time to go through the layers that will help you relax and attempt to witness your thoughts. Witnessing thoughts will help you establish the observer of what is larger than thoughts so you can move beyond them for a truly effective visualization. Get creative and picture allowing your body to rest on the floor while you walk somewhere else, up a hill or stairs, down a hallway, or along a path. If you're visualizing a certain event happening, like nailing that job interview or getting a good night's sleep, go through the process of describing all of your senses, emotions, and thoughts while performing this event. Play it all out as if it were happening in the present moment rather than as if you are seeing it happening in the future. There's more about customizing your Yoga Nidra practice in chapter 12.

Reflect on Your Practice

As your Yoga Nidra practice concludes, give yourself a minute to settle back into your body, roll over to one side, rest in that position for a few moments, and then come back to a seated position. Take a moment to reflect on your practice in your mind. In your Yoga Nidra journal, write down your immediate responses to the practice. Remember to write freely and without edits.

Remember, all parts of your visualization are parts of yourself speaking to your conscious mind. During your visualization, you may encounter an archetype. An archetype is a character or general model for something. Archetypes exist in your unconscious as symbols. For example, often when I tap into the wise person inside of me, it takes the form of Gandalf from *Lord of the Rings*. Gandalf is the archetype of my wise person and helps put a face to something otherwise abstract. I understand that when I visualize Gandalf offering me advice, I'm merely tapping my own deep inner wisdom, which is speaking to my conscious mind. All parts of the vision are parts of myself.

Once during a Yoga Nidra practice, I wanted to hear a message from my wise inner teacher. After fostering a deepening Awareness by going through the steps of my Yoga Nidra practice, like my Sankalpa, Inner Sanctuary, body scan, and so on, to connect to the teacher that resides in my deeper unconscious, I visualized one of my favorite professors from college. We were sitting in his office having a warm chat. I could clearly see all the elements—from the lamp in the corner to the wood grain of his desk. I could hear the chair squeak as he leaned back in thought and stroked his beard. Then he looked at me, almost mischievously out of the corner of his eye, and said, "Whatever you believe in, practice it every day." For me, that visualization was my wise inner teacher reminding me of the importance of practice.

Full Meditation Script

Welcome to Yoga Nidra. Lie down and make yourself as comfortable as possible. Let go of any tension with a sigh.

If you wish to have a Sankalpa, repeat it now as a specific, positive, and present statement of truth. If you wish to use your Inner Sanctuary in this practice, give yourself a moment to fill in the details of your sanctuary using your senses.

Bring your attention to the sensation of your face: your mouth, eyes, ears, and nose. Feel your scalp: the top of your head and back of your head. Feel your face and scalp simultaneously. Feel your entire head. Feel the sensation of your neck and throat. Your collarbones and chest. Feel your arms: shoulders, elbows, forearms, wrists, and hands. Feel only the left arm, only the right arm. Left. Right. Feel both arms. While sensations change, they reveal that which is never changing: Awareness. Be Awareness itself. As Awareness, experience yourself as belly, back. Now feel your pelvis. Feel your legs. Feel your feet. Feel your entire body as sensation. Feel your entire body. Sensations may change, but Awareness never does. Be Awareness. Relax a little more than you're relaxed now. Allow your entire body to be relaxed Awareness.

Allow your body to rest on the floor and take an inner journey down a hallway. You can feel your arms and legs moving as you walk deeper and deeper down the hallway. You can see the hallway. You hear the sound of your footsteps as you move farther and farther down the hallway. You know that you're on a journey to see a very wise person. This person has an important message for you. The message will come to you when the time is right.

As you're walking down the hallway, there's a door off to your left. As you open the door, you see a small room with a screen projecting all of your thoughts. Notice your thoughts. Invite, acknowledge, and observe thinking. There's nothing to control; you're merely witnessing thoughts. Then close the door and walk farther down the hallway.

At the end of the hallway, there's a beautiful door. As you approach the door, notice what the door looks like. As you open the door, there's a wise person there waiting for you in the room. Who is the wisest person you can think of in this moment? This person can be real or imagined, living or passed on, old or young. This wise person knows and loves you. This person knows your successes and mistakes. This wise person knows you so well that they could predict your future. This person knows you perhaps even better than you know yourself.

With a wide smile, this wise person welcomes you into this beautiful room and invites you to sit down. This person says that there is something very important about you that they need to tell you. It will be the first thing in your mind. Don't try to think or create anything. It will come on its own. Your wise person says to you, "The very important thing about you that I wanted to tell you is . . ." Hear the first thing that comes to you. Pause for a moment and wait for the words to come. Perhaps it comes in words, a feeling, thought, emotion, or image. Maybe the message will come minutes, hours, or days later, but it will come.

With a broad smile and a hug, this wise person says goodbye. You head back out the door and back up the way you came. You can come back whenever you like. You return up the hallway with the gift of the wise person's message in your heart.

Feel your body walking back up the hallway, closer and closer to the place you came from. For a moment, you check in with the room that has your thoughts on the screen. They are still moving. You close the door again and continue up the hallway until you feel your body lying on the floor.

Feel your body lying on the floor. Remember your Sankalpa and Inner Sanctuary if you used them and remember the wise person's message.

When you hear me count down from five (or ring the bell), that will signal the end of the Yoga Nidra practice.

5, 4, 3, 2, 1 (or ring the bell).

Yoga Nidra is over.

CHAPTER ELEVEN

STEP 10: INTEGRATE YOUR PRACTICE

How to Integrate the Full Yoga Nidra Practice

The final step in the 10-step process is to integrate all 10 steps into one seamless whole. This will be a longer, more complete Yoga Nidra practice where you will experience each of the 10 steps in one practice. The end result will be to experience a richer, deeper, and more integrated experience of Awareness.

Remember, there's no one right way to practice Yoga Nidra. At its essence, Yoga Nidra is about learning to invite, acknowledge, and observe anything that presents itself in your Awareness as a way of learning to identify with your True Nature. It's about becoming Awareness itself. Because there's no right way to practice Yoga Nidra, it can get confusing with the many different approaches to this life-changing practice.

The 10-step method gives you not only the tools to guide you through a Yoga Nidra practice effectively but also the behind-the-scenes information about why those tools are so important. Because you've spent the time learning and practicing each step individually, you'll recognize each leg of the journey like a helpful friend. Not only are each of the 10 steps helpful tools, they are organized in your Yoga Nidra practice as one way of systematically taking you deeper into Awareness. When you put all the practices together, you take the guesswork out of what you might need to have an effective Yoga Nidra practice on any particular day. You also give your body and mind a graduated path to easily relax and open to the experience.

So far along this journey, you've practiced several different Yoga Nidra practices, each one emphasizing different elements of the practice. Each of these practices works as a complete Yoga Nidra experience by itself. You might resonate with one or two individual steps of the practice and therefore might find them as more ready tools to find focus or Awareness, so it's fine, and even encouraged, to listen to any of the other Yoga Nidra practices you've recorded. If you're feeling stuck in an area or just seem to connect to Awareness with body, breath, or mind, for example, do the practices that emphasize those points. If you need a specialized visualization to help you work through or prepare for something, do that practice.

Having said that, I encourage you to do the complete Yoga Nidra practice several times before going back and doing any of the individual practices. Experiencing the full practice will give you a deeper appreciation for each individual step. It will actually strengthen the individual elements of the practice so that if you do need to go back to a particular practice, you'll experience it more deeply.

It's also true that because you've practiced each of the 10 steps individually, you will gain a deeper and quicker state of Awareness in each particular step as you go through the full practice. For this reason, you won't have to spend as much time on each of the steps. Previously, the emphasis for the Yoga Nidra practices in each of the steps was on preparing you for a deep dive into that step. With the complete practice, the emphasis is moving through all of the steps.

What the Full Practice Does for You

Regular Yoga Nidra practice in general, especially doing the full practice, can be truly life-changing. I hope that you have experienced many of the subtle and profound benefits of regularly practicing Yoga Nidra as you've followed the steps of this book. I encourage you to write about the benefits you experience in your Yoga Nidra journal.

The full Yoga Nidra practice is like doing a full-systems checkup regularly for body, mind, and spirit. Practicing regularly will help your entire being operate more smoothly. Your mind will think more clearly and sharply. Your heart will be more open, present with, and in control of your emotions. You'll feel more rested, get better sleep, and feel a vitality and energy animating all your movements. It's not hyperbole that every aspect of your life can improve as a result of Yoga Nidra. I always say that wellness is the by-product of Awareness. As you develop your deepening Awareness through the full Yoga Nidra practice, you'll naturally develop greater wholeness. Living your life from this complete wholeness is perhaps one understanding of enlightenment.

In my own life, Yoga Nidra has shown me more about who I am and about how the Universe works than any other practice. It has helped me experience deep rest and manage fairly acute anxiety. It's given me a beautiful lens of objectivity through which to see life's problems. Knowing my heart's purpose for the world, I see life's problems more for what they are. I'm less reactive, less jealous, and more open to suggestions (just ask my editor).

Yoga Nidra has bolstered my confidence. This practice gives me insight about myself, my teaching, and my business. It has helped me be more creative.

Thanks to Yoga Nidra, I've had some really vivid dreams, visions, and personal insight. It's helped me notice the smallest details of this life with delight. It's helped me to be more present as a husband and father, friend, and family member. It has helped me heal from years of emotional repression. It taught me that emotions are a beautiful and welcome part of my human experience. Yoga Nidra opens me to feel the love that is coursing through me at all times. The residual feeling I get most commonly after Yoga Nidra is one of a sustained love for myself and the world. It's opened up my heart and whispered to me my heart's gifts for the world and shown me ways that I can share them with the world. Indeed, this book is one of the myriad manifestations of my Yoga Nidra practice.

And just like Yoga Nidra practice has helped me along life's journey, the full Yoga Nidra practice is designed to help you go through all the tools necessary to achieve Awareness and effectively move your life in the direction that brings you to wholeness.

10-MINUTE MEDITATION SCRIPT

To begin this Yoga Nidra practice, let out a few deep sighs to release any tension. Invite, acknowledge, and observe everything that comes into your Awareness.

Create your Sankalpa and repeat it in your head a few times. Now establish your Inner Sanctuary.

Bring your attention to the sensation of your face: your mouth, eyes, ears, and nose. Feel your scalp: the top of your head and back of your head. Feel your face and scalp simultaneously. Feel your entire head. Feel the sensation of your neck and throat. Your collarbones and chest. Feel your arms: shoulders, elbows, forearms, wrists, and hands. Feel only left arm, only right arm. Left. Right. Feel both arms. Experience yourself as belly, as back. Now feel your pelvis, your legs, your feet. Feel your entire body as sensation. Feel your entire body. Sensations may change, but Awareness never does. Be Awareness.

Notice your breath. Notice how you feel energy in your body. Choose a part of your body that feels alive. Now choose a part that feels weak or tired. Feel aliveness. Feel low energy. Now feel both energies simultaneously. Though energy changes, Awareness is constant.

Notice any emotion present in this moment. Simply invite, acknowledge, and observe the emotion. Go to your Inner Sanctuary if an emotion is too difficult. What is the opposite of that emotion? What does that emotion feel like? Now feel both emotions. Though you have emotions, you are much larger than emotions. Be Awareness.

Notice your thoughts. Are they moving fast or slow? Simply notice your thoughts. Remember what it feels like to be sharp and focused. Remember what it feels like to feel confused. Sharp and focused. Confused. Now feel both. Be the Awareness that watches your thoughts.

Now remember feeling happy, loving, or sensual. Using your senses, bring a scene of happiness, love, or sensuality to life in this moment. What does happiness, love, or sensuality feel like in your body? Now let go of the scene and simply rest in the feeling in your body in this moment. This feeling always exists. It's your natural way of being.

Visualize yourself walking down a path in the forest. Animal messengers will greet you on your path. They can either speak or communicate directly with your mind. As you turn a corner, there's a large deer. What does the deer say? Continue to move down your path. There is a log that has fallen on the path long ago, upon which is a beaver. What does the beaver say?

You now decide to rest by lying down. As you look up into the sky, you see an eagle. The eagle lands on a branch nearby. What does the eagle say? Now continue along your path and realize that you've made a large circle and you're back to where you started. Remember what your messengers told you.

As the observer, notice yourself having the experience of practicing Yoga Nidra. Remember the feeling of happiness, love, or sensuality you feel, which is always very close to your surface. Observe your thoughts. Observe your emotions. Observe energy and breath in your body. Notice the feeling of your body lying on the floor.

For a brief moment, remember your Inner Sanctuary. Repeat the messages from your messengers. Repeat your Sankalpa.

When you hear me count down from five (or ring the bell), that will signal the end of the Yoga Nidra practice. Because of the work that you've done today in your full Yoga Nidra practice, you'll go back out into your life feeling more alive, happy, and genuine.

5, 4, 3, 2, 1 (or ring the bell).

Yoga Nidra is over.

Get Started

Record either the short or long meditation (or both) in this chapter. As always, prepare for your full Yoga Nidra practice by setting a time and a place that is likely to help you have the most success, a time when you will be alert and undisturbed. Know that a full Yoga Nidra practice will likely take longer than the other Yoga Nidra practices you've been doing. The long meditation script may take 25 to 35 minutes. Make any necessary preparations, including arranging your Yoga Nidra nest and having your journal ready.

Because this practice takes a little longer, also be sure to take care of your bio needs (liquid in, liquid out).

Begin with any of the sensory, movement, mindfulness, or breathing exercises you've learned previously, such as:

⊘ Going on a "sensory safari" through your house (page 29).

⊘ Some gentle yoga postures (page 50).

⊘ Breathing exercises like Ujjayi Breath (page 46) or Bhramari Breath (page 96).

⊘ The countdown meditation (page 51) or "There Is" meditation (page 73).

⊘ Emotional awareness exercise with pictures (page 62).

For this longer practice, it's nice to give yourself a little extra cushion. I like to add one more blanket folded longways on my yoga mat. Some people keep a blowup mattress handy to use for longer Yoga Nidra practices. While not quite as sleep-inducing as a regular mattress, a blowup mattress might be more comfortable than lying on the floor for an extended period of time, especially if the floor is hard.

A longer Yoga Nidra practice means deeper Awareness and deeper relaxation. If deeper relaxation causes you to fall asleep, don't lose sleep over it. Relaxed Awareness is what you are aiming for. If you can stay awake, great; it's nice to remember your experience, but the part of you that receives the benefit is larger than your waking consciousness. Falling asleep is both the product of your body's natural relaxation mechanism as well as the fact that sometimes, with deeper Awareness, the conscious mind can't comprehend the level of work and therefore shuts down into sleep. The part of you that is paying attention to the Yoga Nidra practice does so regardless if you're awake or asleep.

This is as good a time as any to mention ideas for good sleep hygiene. If you find that you fall asleep every or almost every time you practice Yoga Nidra, either you're doing some extremely profound work on your mat or you're simply not getting enough regular, good sleep. Some ideas for good sleep hygiene could include:

⫘ Adopting a regular sleep schedule (this is essential).

⫘ Avoiding caffeine, especially seven hours before bedtime.

⫘ Avoiding blue lights, computer screens, smartphones, and LED lights for at least an hour before bed.

⫘ Giving yourself time to wind down with maybe some light yoga poses, breathing exercises, a bath, and light reading before bedtime.

⫘ Going to bed visualizing your Inner Sanctuary or doing the countdown meditation to relax your mind by allowing it to think of something simple and positive rather than dropping into a sinkhole of worry.

Many people love to do Yoga Nidra to fall asleep. Personally, I avoid doing Yoga Nidra as a way of falling asleep because for me I feel it trains me to sleep during Yoga Nidra. Plus, I feel it messes with my sleep—it tends to keep me in that transitional state between waking and dreaming all night long, or for several hours. Other people love to fall asleep with Yoga Nidra. You can try it for yourself and see whether or not it works for you.

The last note before jumping into the full practice is to let go of all expectations and simply agree to invite, acknowledge, and observe (maybe respond) to whatever presents itself to you.

Reflect on Your Practice

As your full Yoga Nidra practice concludes, give yourself a moment to come back into your body. Remember what time of day it is and what you've been doing—especially if you found yourself in a sense of timelessness. Eventually, roll over to one side and rest in that position for a few moments. When you're ready, make your way up to a seated position. Repeat your Sankalpa to yourself.

In your Yoga Nidra journal, write down your immediate responses to the practice. As usual, just get the words onto the page without editing yourself. You can also respond to some or all of these questions in your journal:

🖋 What was your Sankalpa?

🖋 How was doing a full Yoga Nidra practice different from other practices?

🖋 What part(s) of the practice in particular stood out to you as effective or powerful?

🖋 Do certain steps feel more difficult than others? If so, why?

🖋 Did you experience relaxation during the full Yoga Nidra practice? What was it like?

🖋 How much of the practice do you remember?

🖋 Did anything unexpected arise during your practice? If so, what was it?

🖋 Did you gain any particular insight, images, or direction during your practice?

✐ Did you encounter, think of, or receive anything you could expand on, investigate, or meditate upon in waking life? If so, what and how?

Remember that your practice will evolve the more you do it. If you fell asleep or if nothing really spectacular happened, that's fine. Spectacular isn't the goal. If you did have a spectacular experience, wonderful! Still, that's not the goal. Awareness is. Simply notice your experience and write down what happened (it can be fascinating to track your experiences this way). Whatever occurred, try to avoid having expectations for future practices.

Though you have been building up to this point in your knowledge and practice of Yoga Nidra, the full practice represents simply putting all of the pieces together for a deeper experience. Also consider that the practice works on a level you may be unaware of in the moment but which might manifest the more you do it. No matter what kind of experience you had, I invite you to commit to doing this practice at least once a day for five days to explore how your experience of it changes over the course of those five days. Do the long version if possible, but short's okay if you're short on time.

Quite often after a full Yoga Nidra practice, I'll feel a lightness in my being that is unparalleled in my everyday sensory experience. I often feel a sense of peace, love, and acceptance with the world. After a full practice, it seems as if everything makes sense even though I don't have all the answers to life's questions and problems. This experience feels like coming home. Then a beautiful new practice emerges, the practice of living my everyday life from this place of deep calm, love, and Awareness. The practice of living and acting from Awareness is as rewarding as it is challenging. And like every practice, the more I do it the better I get. Somehow, even in this practice is the invitation to become ever more Aware. Somehow in this practice, I'm revealing to my conscious mind how I'm supposed to be.

Full Meditation Script

Welcome to Yoga Nidra. Lie down and make yourself as comfortable as possible. Begin your full Yoga Nidra practice with a few deep sighs to release any tension. Your only work is to invite, acknowledge, and observe anything and everything that comes into your Awareness.

Now, create your Sankalpa with a phrase that is positive, specific, and present, such as "I'm on the road toward . . ." and fill in the blank or "I have everything inside of me for . . ." and fill in the blank. Once you've decided on your Sankalpa, repeat it in your head a few times. This plants a seed of intention deep in your Awareness.

Next, establish your Inner Sanctuary, your personal safe haven, by visualizing a place that you either remember or can imagine. Fill in the details of this place using your senses. You can come back to this sanctuary anytime you wish.

In this moment, feel the sensation of your body lying on the floor. Feel your entire body. Feel the entire front side of your body. Now the back side. Now feel your entire body, front and back. Invite, acknowledge, and observe the feeling of your body on the floor. Now bring your attention to the sensation of your mouth. Bring your attention to your eyes. Now feel your ears. Feel your entire face: your forehead, eyebrows, eyes, bridge of your nose and nostrils, cheekbones, upper lip, lower lip, chin, and jaw. Feel your entire face.

Now notice the sensation of the crown of your head. Feel the back of your head. Feel your entire scalp, your crown, and the back of your head. Now feel your entire head at the same time. Now bring your attention to the sensation of your arms, your chest, and collarbones. Feel your belly and notice it as it breathes. Feel the sensation of your back on the floor. Feel your entire back. As Awareness, bring your attention to the sensation of your pelvis. Feel your entire pelvis as sensation. Now feel your legs from hips to toes. Feel both legs from hips to toes. Feel only the left leg. Feel only the right leg. Left. Right. Feel both legs.

Feel your entire body lying on the floor. What's aware of the body lying on the floor? Notice what is observing the body lying on the floor. Be unchanging Awareness. Without trying to control or do anything, simply notice your level of relaxation. If there's any way you can relax more, do so.

As Awareness, notice your breath. Notice how you feel energy in your body at this moment. Choose a part of your body that feels alive with vitality. Describe to yourself how this energy feels in your body. Now choose a part of your body that feels low-energy, weak, or tired. Describe it to yourself. Feel the part of your body with the vital energy. Now bring your attention to only the part that feels low-energy. Now feel both energies at the same time. Feel both at the same time. Energy is always changing. Though energy changes, your Awareness is constant.

As Awareness, notice which emotion you have in this moment or which emotion you've been working with lately. Simply invite, acknowledge, and observe the emotion. No need to fix or change it. If ever an emotion gets too difficult to work with, go back to your Inner Sanctuary. Where do you feel that emotion? If this emotion could speak, what would it say to you? Now what is its opposite emotion? What does that feel like? Release that emotion and go back to the first emotion. Now release the first emotion and go back to the opposite emotion. Now feel both emotions. What is the part of you that is large enough to hold both emotions simultaneously? Simply witness emotions. You have emotions, but you are larger than emotions. Be Awareness itself.

As Awareness, notice your thoughts. Don't control or change them. Are your thoughts moving fast or slow? What is the subject of your thoughts? Notice if your thoughts evoke memories, other thoughts, words, or emotions. Now remember what it feels like to be sharp and focused in your thoughts. Now remember what it feels like to feel muddy or confused in your thoughts. Sharp and focused. Muddy. Now feel both, like you could think very clearly about one thing and be very confused about another. Observe your thinking mind. Though you have thoughts, you are much larger than thoughts.

Now using your senses, remember a time when you felt very happy, loving, or sensual. What does happiness, love, or sensuality feel like in your body? Is there a particular part of your body that feels that emotion or sensation? Allow that feeling to spread into every part of your body and beyond, as if your body weren't large enough to contain all the happiness, love, or sensuality you're feeling in this moment. Now let go of the memories and simply rest in the feeling in your body in this moment. What is feeling, experiencing, and witnessing this feeling? This feeling was there all along. You don't need anything to feel this; it's your natural way of being. Feel free in this happiness, love, or sensuality. This is you.

As Awareness, observe yourself lying on the floor having this Yoga Nidra experience. Notice all the parts working together from body to energy to thoughts to emotions—and all the rest. You're simply witnessing yourself lying on the floor having this experience. It's all happening in this moment.

Now visualize yourself walking down a small path in the forest. See the sunlight through the trees. Hear the sound of the wind and birds. Your feet are connecting to the soft earth. Feel the sun on your skin and smell the pine trees and wildflowers. There are a few animal messengers you will see on your journey who can either speak or communicate directly to your mind. You'll recognize their message as the first thing that comes to you.

As you turn a corner, there's a deer standing in your path. What does the deer say? Pause for a moment and hear the deer. Thank the deer and continue along your way. Continue to move down your path. There is a log that has fallen long ago over the path. As you are stepping over the log, you see a beaver. What does the beaver say? Hear the beaver. Thank the beaver and continue along your way. You decide to rest by lying down in the grass on the side of the path. As you look up into the sky, you see a large eagle soaring in the clouds with its wings spread wide, riding the currents. The eagle flies toward you and lands on a nearby branch. What does the eagle say? Hear the eagle. Thank the eagle. Feeling rested, continue your journey and realize that you've made a large circle. You're back to where you started. Give yourself a moment and repeat the messages of the deer, the beaver, and the eagle. The visualization is finished.

As the observer, notice yourself having the experience of practicing Yoga Nidra. Remember the feeling of happiness, love, or sensuality you feel, which is always very close to your surface. Observe your thoughts without any opinion about them. You're simply noticing thoughts. Observe your emotions. Simply observe emotions. Now observe energy and breath in your body. Notice the feeling of your body lying on the floor. Pay particular attention to the feeling of the soles of your feet and the palms of your hands. Notice the feeling of your belly. Bring yourself to feel the sensation of your entire body.

For a brief moment, revisit your Inner Sanctuary and feel all of your senses. Repeat the messages from your messengers one more time. Repeat your Sankalpa.

When you hear me count down from five (or ring the bell), that will signal the end of the Yoga Nidra practice. Because of the work that you've done today in your full Yoga Nidra practice, you'll go back out into your life feeling more alive, happy, and genuine. You'll feel in touch with the deepest parts of yourself. You'll move through your life with wisdom and wonder.

5, 4, 3, 2, 1 (or ring the bell).

Yoga Nidra is over.

CHAPTER TWELVE

STRENGTHENING YOUR YOGA NIDRA PRACTICE

Welcome to Inner Peace

You made it! You are now a practitioner of the ancient, transformative practice of Yoga Nidra. Now it's time to create a sustainable Yoga Nidra practice so you can continue to reap the benefits for years to come.

I've mentioned this a dozen times, and here's lucky number 13: This is a practice. The point in practice is just to show up and do it. That's it. Naturally, you'll learn more about Yoga Nidra as you practice it, and naturally you'll get better and better at developing your Awareness, but the point of the practice is to regularly step up to your edge, your frontier of

Awareness through your human experience. I say all this to say, release your ambitions of the practice. Let go of the idea of mastering Yoga Nidra. Instead, allow the practice of Yoga Nidra to master you. Allow the experience to unfold in exactly the way it does and agree to simply invite, acknowledge, and observe. That's all.

Of course it is useful and, in fact, beneficial to use your Sankalpa as a compass, a guiding star that will inform your unfolding, but that's very different from holding expectations for the practice. Having an ambition to become enlightened, to uncover and heal your deepest wounds, or to turn into a superhuman overnight will certainly leave you feeling disappointed.

Many times you've put your order in to the Universe with your Sankalpa and you wait around for it to manifest, but it never seems to come. It's like you've ordered your Sankalpa online and you're staying at home all day waiting for the FedEx delivery person to show up and hand the results to you. You keep ignoring the doorbell because the UPS delivery person shows up instead of FedEx. Eventually you realize that though the delivery person might have a different uniform than you expected, you are still being delivered what you ordered.

Stay open to whatever presents itself. Everything is the messenger, even and especially if it doesn't come in the form you expected. In part, Yoga Nidra gives us the Awareness to discern when we've received what we were looking for.

Jazz artist Louis Armstrong said, "What we play is life." And, ultimately, it's life that we're practicing. We practice welcoming, recognizing, witnessing, and sometimes responding to every thought, emotion, and experience. Your Yoga Nidra practice is the best way that I know of learning to do exactly this. As you continue to practice Yoga Nidra, those who spend the most time with you will begin to notice something different about you. You might simply tell them that you've been sleeping better.

Customizing Your Practice

Now that you've taken the full tour of Yoga Nidra's 10 steps, you can start to customize how you practice or which Yoga Nidra practices you do to help you be most effective in your practice. You might begin by reviewing your Yoga Nidra journal to notice those things that really jump out at you.

What was the best time of day for you to practice? Choosing the best time of day for you to practice is key for getting the most out of the practice. I've noticed that doing Yoga Nidra first thing in the morning or later in the evening before going to sleep is less productive than, say, midmorning or afternoon. My mind is much more alert during these times, so I can get into a state of relaxed Awareness much easier than I would in the early morning or later evening when I usually just fall asleep. Since you've been practicing regularly, it's likely you have a good idea what your best times are, too.

What were your favorite parts of Yoga Nidra practice? There's no value in practicing Yoga Nidra one way over the other. As always, you're simply practicing Awareness. Whether that's the full practice, the joy practice, or the body scan practice, each one will help you cultivate Awareness. Choose the practice that works best for you and do that one regularly.

Did any parts of any of the practices stir up any strong emotions? These could be messengers that are most important to you. Remember that sometimes an emotion is a call to action, and these messengers are inviting you to respond in a particular way to continue growing in your life.

Was there any meditation that was particularly soothing? Having a few practices in your back pocket that you know will help calm you after a long or hectic day might be useful.

Can you make your Yoga Nidra practice part of your cooldown routine for your regular exercise regimen? I love to trail run, and once, after a nice long run, I took several minutes to cool down with some yoga stretches on the grass. Then I lay down and led myself through a Yoga Nidra practice (yes, you can do Yoga Nidra anywhere, even without all the props). In that practice, my body became relaxed and my mind became alert. I had a vision of a Native American elder who told me, "Your ancestors are on the table." The elder then beat a drum, which caused me to bolt upright. This message led me on a fascinating journey of learning more about some of my ancestors. About a week later, I wasn't surprised when I visited my dad and on his table was a book of genealogy complete with photos and letters.

Customizing Your Yoga Nidra Script

As you familiarize yourself with the full practice presented in chapter 11 and see how the parts work together and recognize the parts you need most or tend to find easiest to work with, you may wish to write your own scripts. Since you know what you need better than anyone, you are fully equipped to create a Yoga Nidra practice customized just for you. Simply follow the 10 steps through this basic format:

1. Yoga Nidra prep: Set up your nest; do sensory, movement, mindfulness, or breathing exercises; get comfortable, close your eyes, and release tension with a sigh.

2. Go through the 10 steps, starting with your Sankalpa.

3. Spend the last few minutes retracing your steps back through the 10 steps.

4. Make a definitive end to your practice by either counting down from five or ringing a bell.

If you want to focus on one of the steps rather than going through a full practice, follow this format:

1. Yoga Nidra prep: Set up your nest; do sensory, movement, mindfulness, or breathing exercises; get comfortable, close your eyes, and release tension with a sigh.

2. Go through the first three steps: Sankalpa, Inner Sanctuary, and body scan (long or short, depending on how much focus you want to give this).

3. Jump to any step you wish or progress through the other steps quickly until you get to the step you want to focus on.

4. Spend the last few minutes of your practice retracing your steps back through the steps you traveled.

5. Make a definitive end to your practice by either counting down from five or ringing a bell.

Whichever way you practice, as you go through the practice, make sure that once in a while you play with opposites as separate things and then ask yourself to become aware of them simultaneously, as you learned to do in step 8 (for example, feeling frustration, then feeling peace, then frustration, then peace, then both). You can play with opposites in any of the steps from body scan through visualization. Playing with opposites is a valuable and simple tool to help you move deeper into Awareness in all of the steps. Hopefully you've experienced this deepening as you've followed the scripts in this book.

After each practice, ground yourself by pausing for a brief moment and connecting to body, time of day, and so on. Our Both/And nature invites us to live this life with Awareness in a way that is mindful and practical rather than floating in a realm above it. Sometimes after a particularly deep practice, if my mind feels like it's floating in the clouds, I'll take a moment to connect with my body with a few yoga poses or breathing exercises to become grounded and focused on important and practical things like driving my car and picking up my kid.

Eventually, you'll be good enough at building your own custom Yoga Nidra practice that you will be able to lead yourself through Yoga Nidra without a script. You'll notice a curious thing about your thinking mind, which is building the practice for you as you go along while your Awareness is simply watching the whole thing transpire. This is a beautiful way that the mind and Awareness can work in harmony rather than against each other and to truly practice your Both/And nature.

To lead yourself through a practice without a recording, simply go through the steps in your mind. Be curious about those things that pop into your Awareness and simply invite, acknowledge, and observe them as they do. Either keep your Awareness on whatever presents itself or move along the process through the 10 steps. This is a little different from a mindfulness meditation exercise in that you still have the basic format for Yoga Nidra, including your Sankalpa, Inner Sanctuary, and deepening layers of Awareness.

Carrying Your Practice Forward

Nothing helps us progress like developing good habits. Choose a few times a week or a particular time every day to practice Yoga Nidra regularly so it becomes one of your healthiest habits. Hopefully by now I don't have to tell you how beneficial it is for you. Keep your Yoga Nidra journal handy and reflect often on the things you notice as you practice. Periodically, go back and notice what was percolating in your Awareness during your practice weeks or months prior. It might help you notice your evolving Awareness.

Keep your practice flexible. Do it as often as you can fit it in. You can always vary the time of day, place you practice, and which script you use. Especially if you've recorded all of the scripts on your phone, you can easily take a moment when you have a break during the day and close your eyes and listen.

I also encourage you to find Yoga Nidra classes in your area, ask your regular yoga teacher about the practice, and find some teachers and practices online that you might resonate with. I have dozens of classes on my website that I've recorded, which are free and available for all. I also suggest a wonderful free meditation app called Insight Timer. There are literally thousands of Yoga Nidra recordings that you can listen to. (See the resources section on page 136.)

I hope you've found this book helpful and that it will be an ongoing resource for you. It's been an honor to be with you on this Yoga Nidra journey, and I wish you well on the next phase of your personal journey. I'd like to end with this . . .

For me, Yoga Nidra has become a beautiful practice of Awareness. Even when I'm teaching it, I experience the same levels of deepening Awareness as if I were lying on the floor and practicing. One day after a heart-expanding Yoga Nidra class in Manhattan, I found myself walking down Amsterdam Avenue on my way back to the subway to catch the 2,3 line to Brooklyn. The practice I'd just led had quickened my body, mind, and spirit with a calm and satisfying love, and it was like my entire world opened up.

My vision was clear, and I felt as though I could see every detail of every bird, and as I looked down Amsterdam Avenue, I could see for miles, all the way downtown to the Hudson River. I could hear the happy chirping of the birds and swish of cars as they passed, all with astounding clarity. As each person passed me on the street, I could feel into their heart. Whether the person was scowling, smiling, or neither, each person I passed felt like pure love. Suddenly, somehow everything, every person, object, and animal—even the rats in the subway station—were all boiled down to a pure expression of love. The entire Universe was a positive affirmation of existence. That clarion moment helped me understand three essential truths: Love is everything. Everything is YES! It's all so simple.

May love be our eternal practice.

Resources

Insight Timer app: insighttimer.com (https://insighttimer.com /scottmooreyoga)

iRest with Dr. Richard Miller: www.irest.org/users/richard-c-miller

Scott Moore Yoga: www.scottmooreyoga.com. Yoga Nidra recordings: www.scottmooreyoga.com/yoga-nidra-recordings

Scott Moore YouTube channel: "SYTP Module 1." *YouTube* video, 8:25 (www.youtube.com/watch?v=WDgFW-NfyJE)

ParaYoga (Yoga Nidra with Rod Stryker): www.parayoga.com

An Interview with Dr. Richard Miller: Buddha at the Gas Pump. "Richard Miller—Buddha at the Gas Pump Interview." *YouTube* video, 2:29:01. www.youtube.com/watch?v=dSfGFoy8Ltc.

References

Beard, Allison. "Life's Work: An Interview with Greg Louganis." *Harvard Business Review*. Accessed August 13, 2019. hbr.org/2016/07/lifes-work-an-interview-with-greg-louganis.

Bergland, Christopher. "The Neuroscience of Perseverance: Dopamine Reinforces the Habit of Perseverance." *Psychology Today*. December 6, 2011. Accessed August 12, 2019. www.psychologytoday.com/us/blog/the-athletes-way/201112/the-neuroscience-perseverance.

Farhi, Donna. *Bringing Yoga to Life: The Everyday Practice of Enlightened Living*. New York, NY: HarperCollins Publishers, 2005.

Gustafson, Craig. "Bruce Lipton, PhD: The Jump From Cell Culture to Consciousness." *Integrative Medicine: A Clinician's Journal* 16, no. 6 (December 2017): 44. www.ncbi.nlm.nih.gov/pmc/articles/PMC6438088/.

Moore, Scott. "Stress Relief with Yoga Nidra." *Conscious Life News*. September 9, 2018. Accessed August 12, 2019. https://consciouslifenews.com/stress-relief-yoga-nidra/11136776/.

Rani, K., S. C. Tiwari, S. Kumar, U. Singh, J. Prakash, and N. Srivastava. "Psycho-Biological Changes with Add on Yoga Nidra in Patients with Menstrual Disorders: A Randomized Clinical Trial." *Journal of Caring Sciences* 5, no. 1 (March 2016): 1–9. DOI:10.15171/jcs.2016.001.

Schacter, D. L., D. R. Addis, D. Hassabis, V. C. Martin, R. N. Spreng, and K. K. Szpunar. The future of memory: remembering, imagining, and the brain. *Neuron*, 76(4) (2012), 677–694.

Scott Moore Yoga. "How to Relieve Stress: Sourcing Your True Power by Being Stress Free." Accessed August 12, 2019. www.scottmooreyoga.com/how-to-relieve-stress.

Whyte, David. *Clear Mind, Wild Heart*. Audio CD. Louisville, CO; Sounds True, 2002.

Index

A

Adrenaline, 26

Ali, Muhammad, 105

Annamaya kosha, 37

Anandamaya kosha (bliss body), 83

Annamaya kosha (body layer), 59

"Anthem" (Cohen), 15

Armstrong, Louis, 130

Asana, 95

Awareness, 1–6

body scan, 35–36

breath, 45, 48

emotions, 59, 62

integrating experience of, 113–116

relaxed, 1, 5–6, 17, 37, 50, 93, 110,
    119, 131

safe haven, 23, 25

Self-observation, 91, 93

tapping into joy, 85, 88

visualization, 103–105

witnessing thoughts, 70–74

Yoga Nidra philosophy, 14

B

Ballet West, 2

Bhramari Breath, 96, 119

Body scan, 4, 35

benefits of, 37

five (5)-minute meditation script,
    38–39

full meditation script, 42–43

getting started, 39–40

how to do a, 35–36

journaling in reflection, 40–42

Brain, interpreting information, 25–26

Breath

Bhramari Breath, 96, 119

benefits of practice, 46–48

Bumblebee Breath, 96

countdown meditation, 51, 119, 120

five (5)-minute meditation script,
    48–49

full meditation script, 53–55

getting started, 49–51

how to tune in to breath, 45–46

journaling practice, 51–52

Prana (energy), 47

Ujjayi Breath, 46, 49, 50–51, 53, 63,
    96, 119

Victorious Breath, 46

Whisper Breath, 46

yoga poses, 49–50

Bringing Yoga to Life (Farhi), 14

Bumblebee Breath, 96

C

Carrey, Jim, 105

Clear Mind, Wild Heart (audio
    program), 82

Cohen, Leonard, 15

Comfort, 6

Corpse pose, Savasana, 5–6

Cortisol, 26

Acknowledgments

I'm immensely grateful for my wife and son, who supported me while I holed up to write this book. Thank you to all my teachers, namely Dr. Richard Miller, Rod Stryker, Donna Farhi, Erin Geesaman-Rabke, Peter Francyk, Judith Lasater, Schuyler Grant, Matt Phippen, Jaisri Lambert, Chris Tompkins, Drs. Suma and Sathyanarayanan, and Tita Juanito. Thanks to the inimitable support of family, namely my loving parents; my twin brother, Chris; and my sister, Lucy. Thanks to Laurel, Greg, Liam and Lucy, Kim, John, Nan, Garrick, Jason, Merit, and Christy.

About the Author

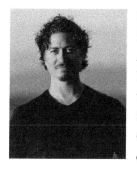

Scott Moore (E-RYT 500) has been teaching yoga and mindfulness since 2003. A former owner of two yoga studios, he loves teaching at retreats, at workshops, at teacher trainings, and in virtual classrooms. Scott was a professor at Westminster College for nine years and developed the curriculum for accredited courses for Yoga for Wellness. More than 30,000 people have listened to his Yoga Nidra recordings on the app Insight Timer. He also writes for and has been featured in *Yoga Journal, Conscious Life News, Elephant Journal, Mantra Wellness, Medium,* and his own blog at www.scottmooreyoga.com. He lives in Southern France and loves to travel the world with his wife and son.

CPSIA information can be obtained
at www.ICGtesting.com
Printed in the USA
BVHW091430121219
566019BV00002B/3/P